AF886153

Basic Guide to Veterinary Hospital Management

 First edition 1992.
Printed in the U.S.A.

ISBN: 0-941451-51-8

TABLE OF CONTENTS

PREFACE TO THE SECOND EDITION

The second edition of the book comes as the result of the encouragement and support of many people. First, the committees, Board of Directors, and staff of the American Animal Hospital Association, especially Marilyn Bergquist and Debby Morehead, who have published and marketed the book and made it a success. Secondly, those who bought the first edition and especially those who have made suggestions as to how to improve it. I give special thanks to Margaret Banks, financial administrator of the Oradell Animal Hospital in Oradell, New Jersey, and Tammy Fritts, hospital administrator of the Veterinary Medical Center in Tulsa, Oklahoma, who gave me great assistance in developing this second edition. I also thank Mr. Sheldon I. London Esq., author of *How to Comply With Federal Employee Laws*, for his and his wonderful book's assistance in the new section on those laws. My special thanks is saved for my good friend Dr. Bob Featherston of Tulsa, Oklahoma, who wrote the entire new chapter in this edition on "Computer Use in Veterinary Hospital Management." Besides being a very busy practitioner, Dr. Featherston has become one of veterinary medicine's foremost experts on computer use. Thank you, Bob. You are the true definition of a friend.

To my new readers: I welcome your comments, criticisms, and suggestions. They will help me with the third edition.

John B. McCarthy, DVM, MBA
May 1995

PREFACE

The purpose of this manual is to provide a useable guidebook for the management of animal hospitals. While there is no real new or original material in this manual, to my knowledge this is the first time all this information has been included in one publication. That is the distinction of this manual. Because of this distinction, this manual should be an invaluable aid to anyone who has the responsibility of managing an animal hospital, whether you are experienced or a novice, owner or nonowner, veterinarian or nonveterinarian, teacher or student. The manual is not meant to be read as a novel but to be used as a reference when a given situation or problem arises. It is also designed as a teaching guide for new employees or for students. I have tried not to be judgmental but to give alternative courses in most situations—especially concerning computers. I am not an attorney or an accountant and advise that you ask the advice of the appropriate professional in those cases where the condition warrants that advice.

The appendices should be most helpful to the animal hospital manager, as they are an assortment of sample forms and information sources to supplement the text. This assortment is by no means all-inclusive. It is meant to show the variety of available materials. I encourage you to search out the additional sources of management information listed in Appendix A and become students of management.

I thank all who have studied this subject before me and whose work I have referenced. I thank the American Animal Hospital Association for giving me the stimulus over 20 years ago to recognize the need for animal hospital management education as well as their willingness to publish this manual. I thank my partners, employees, and clients of my former animal hospital who allowed me to practice most of what I preached for 25 years. I thank the instructors in my courses at Long Island University for the stimulation that they have given me to become a student of management, and I especially thank my wife, Ruth, and my family for their support in my endeavors and for the hours that I could have been with them but wasn't.

John B. McCarthy, DVM, MBA
October 1991

Chapter 1

MANAGEMENT INFORMATION: WHY YOU NEED IT AND WHERE TO GET IT

Why You Need It

The major pitfalls in managing a small business, as reported to Dun and Bradstreet by people who are actually in business, are lack of experience, lack of money, the wrong location, inventory mismanagement, too much capital going into fixed assets, poor credit-granting practices, taking too much out for yourself, unplanned expansion, or having the wrong attitude.[1]

As a manager of an animal hospital, you are responsible for the success of that business. You must always consider that the animal hospital must be run as a business. In spite of all the wonderful, modern medical care that patients may receive, the business will not survive poor or absent management.

All basic management rules are totally applicable to your situation. As the list above suggests, the most common reasons for failure of a business are poor management and poor or absent planning.[2] If the business that you are managing is to be successful, you will need management information and skills. You may be sharing the managerial role with the business owners or others, or you may be totally responsible. You should know what your role is and how to fulfill that role. You also should know enough about yourself to know if you are capable of fulfilling that role. You will need to be aware of your own values and your own preferred management style. Without such awareness, you may easily confuse your own sense of what is right or appropriate with what the situation seems to require.[3]

This manual will give you the information and resources you will need to manage an animal hospital as well as help in determining if you have the skills needed to manage. Peter F. Drucker in *The Practice of Management* said, "In a competitive economy, above all, the quality and performance of the managers determine the success of a business, indeed they determine its survival."[4] Your performance as a manager may well determine the success and survival of the animal hospital you are managing.

The Definition of Management

"Management is the art and science of accomplishing the objectives of an organization through the effective and efficient use of others including the determination of the goals."[5] Another simpler way to say this might be "working with and through individuals and groups to accomplish organizational goals."[6] In both cases, the use of the word "organization" refers to the business that you are managing, and also there is a key reference to working with others.

To manage you must not try to do everything yourself. That is not managing. A successful manager knows what needs to be done and accomplishes the goal of getting the task accomplished by others. Managing therefore requires many skills, which will be discussed later, but a special skill, which is a key if the definition of management is to be carried out by the manager, is the skill of leadership.

Leadership occurs anytime anyone attempts to influence the behavior of an individual or group regardless of the reason. Therefore, managing clearly requires that the manager has the ability of leadership, but leadership alone is not managing unless the leadership is directed towards the needs and goals of the business being managed. This is an important concept for you as a manager to understand. Your ability to influence the behavior of others (i.e., get things done) will only be effective and efficient if you are accomplishing the needs and goals of your business. No manager can survive without the ability to lead, but not all leaders are successful managers.[7]

The Management Process

There are four basic parts of the management process. They are all equal in importance; they are present in all managing situations; and the absence of any one can make close attention to the others inconsequential. The four parts are

- **planning**—determining the goals of the business and developing the strategy and tactics to accomplish the goals.
- **organizing**—communicating the plan to those who will be responsible to carry it out and develop the required organization to implement the plan.
- **directing**—personnel management, motivating people, and allocation of resources.
- **control** —determining the success of the management process and providing the information required to determine management decisions.

Not all managers will be equally involved in all parts of the management process. You may have little if anything to do with the planning function and only be asked to organize and direct. The point is that unless there is a planning function carried out (presumably by the business owners), it will be difficult, if not impossible, for you to effectively manage. Any successful business should be goal-oriented rather than procedure-oriented and should have a plan to accomplish those goals. Goals should be realistic and attainable, represent a significant challenge, and represent the philosophy of the owners of the business. The following goals would appear to be realistic and attainable for any animal hospital:

- producing the best possible medical care and service for patients and clients,
- providing reasonable financial return for the owners which will enable the owners to provide reasonable salaries for employees, and
- providing time for the owners to pursue special professional interests, time to devote to organized veterinary medicine and community activities, and time left for personal and family enjoyment.

More specific goals with a target date might be to increase the number of patients seen by 25% in the next six months, or to increase the gross income of the hospital by 30% in the next six months, or to allow the owners to take a one month vacation in the next year.

Whatever the case may be, in order for any business to be properly managed, the person expected to carry out the organizing and directing functions of the management process must have plans and goals to accomplish.

In succeeding chapters, we will discuss the organizing and directing functions of management. The last part of the management process, controlling, asks us to determine how we measure the results of our efforts. Every manager may have a different means to do this; but a general set of measures might be the financial success of the business, the ability of the staff to work as a team, happy, well-motivated employees, or satisfied clients.

Areas of Management in an Animal Hospital

There are five basic management activities involved in managing an animal hospital:

- **personnel management**—hiring, firing, supervising employee activities, and coordinating the work of the professional and support staff.
- **operations and maintenance**—reception of clients and front office management, inventory management, and care of building and equipment.
- **finance**—accounting, bookkeeping, purchasing, debt collections, budgeting, and records control.

- **marketing**—finding and keeping clients and making people aware of a need for the services provided by the hospital that you are managing.
- **community and client relations**—communications with clients and image building.

All of these areas of management will be covered in detail in this manual.

Special Skills of Managers

There are at least three areas of skill that are necessary for carrying out the process of management:

- **technical skill**—your ability to use your knowledge of management as well as your knowledge and familiarity with the equipment, methods, and techniques used in the hospital.
- **human skill**—understanding the people with whom you are working, knowing their past behavior, and being able to predict their future behavior plus understanding what motivates people and being able to effectively lead.
- **conceptual skill**—understanding how well your role fits into the overall operation of the hospital and how the hospital you are managing is affected by its external environment.[8]

Managing an animal hospital can be psychologically and emotionally demanding. Despite the trends toward automation in most industries, real productivity in your business comes primarily from people. Achieving goals for your business will lie in your ability to recognize that human behavior is caused by external stimuli. It will be your responsibility to shape that behavior for productive results. A successful manager also must know the job to be able to manage it. Only then can the manager truly determine how well that job is being done. Any successful manager also will know the boundaries within which to operate. To exceed these boundaries and create problems within the organization will be harmful to all involved.

The most important skill necessary to carry out all areas of management is the ability to communicate. Your ability to communicate will have an affect on everything that you do. You can communicate in the following ways:

- **thinking straight**—this is the first step in good communication. You must have facts and think of what they mean before you do anything else.
- **actions**—you communicate with others by the way you treat them and by your gestures and signs. You communicate by example and how you perform your work.

- **talking**—this is your easiest and most used means of communication but also can be the most dangerous. As your hospital grows and your number of employees becomes larger, you will see that you cannot communicate solely by talking.
- **listening**—this is probably the most overlooked tool of communication. Good listening encourages an adequate flow of information, and it creates a trusting environment and inspires confidence. When you listen, you learn a great deal about people.
- **writing and reading**—this is the most important way that you can communicate in the hospital without having the communication lost, forgotten, or overlooked.[9]

Effective communication devices that are used in well-managed animal hospitals include well-constructed and legible medical records; simple notes to employees, management, or clients with a well-organized and convenient means of distribution such as bulletin boards or mailboxes; personnel policy manual; office and hospital policy manual and booklets; performance evaluations of employees; employee satisfaction surveys; staff meetings; client satisfaction surveys; and computerized messages or computer-generated letters.

Don't depend on a person's memory. Developing good communications as well as communication devices will be your most important management challenge.

How and Where Do I Get the Skills and Information That I Need?

Veterinary medicine is a people business. Not all people relate well to other people. There may be shyness, lack of assertiveness, ability to be easily intimidated, and poor communication skills. Many of these people will not be good managers and should realize that before they start. Some of these traits may be correctable but that should be done before the managing begins. If you accept the responsibility of being a manager, you accept the responsibility of directing, changing, and controlling the behavior of others.[10] If you are not willing to accept that responsibility, you should not attempt to, or be asked to, manage.

The best and most effective way to develop the skills of management is, of course, experience. Experience gained working with or for an experienced manager will offer more than all of the books and magazines ever written on the subject. Knowing and anticipating the pitfalls, as outlined at the beginning of this chapter, can help minimize them. One of the best ways to learn management skills is to study the mistakes of others.[11] Experience, however, is not a uniformly effective teacher. An aphorism criticizes the person who has worked for 20 years but has only reexperienced the first year 20 times. One learns from experience only by testing that experience against tentative generalizations made for the future. Any manager, experienced or not, must always be on the outlook for new ways to do things, for applications of old ideas to new problems, and vice versa. The manager must also be cognizant of laws and regulations affecting the business, especially those pertaining to personnel. A well-versed, successful manager will be familiar with several management-oriented periodicals. There are books that will be very helpful in the art and science of management. The manager should be aware of videotapes and audiotapes for training employees. There also are many opportunities for the manager to attend lectures and workshops on animal hospital-specific topics where they will meet other managers with similar problems to discuss. Appendix A lists several books, periodicals, and sources for videotapes and audiotapes. This list is by no means all inclusive but is meant to offer an opportunity for education and continuing education in management.

References

1. Dennis H. Tootelian and Ralph M. Gaedeke, *Small Business Management*, Scott Foresman and Co., p. 32
2. Ibid, p. 289
3. Priscilla K. Stockner, MS, DVM, MBA, *A Practice Management Manual For Veterinarians*, Stockner and Associates, Chapter 2
4. Peter F. Drucker, *The Practice of Management*, Harper and Row, p. 1
5. John B. Garbarino, MBA, JD, "Management of the Enterprise" (Mgt 501) lecture notes, fall 1984
6. Paul Hersey and Kenneth Blanchard, *Management of Organizational Behavior*, Prentice Hall, fourth edition, p. 3
7. Ibid, p. 3
8. Ibid, p. 5
9. Stockner, Chapter 15
10. Hersey, p. 10
11. Tootelian, p. 32

Chapter 2

PERSONNEL MANAGEMENT

Management Styles and Theories

In the early 1900s, management was only scientific in nature. It was felt that the best way to improve output was to improve techniques and methods used by workers. The manager's function was to set up and enforce performance criteria based on the needs of the organization and not on the needs of the individual.[1] In volume one, number one, of the *Harvard Business Review*, October 1922, Daniel Starch wrote, "Business and industry consist in the control of human beings who in turn control the physical forces, materials and machines and in that broad sense business is psychological in nature."[2] In the 1920s and 1930s, the human relations movement entered the management arena.[3] Since then, much has been written and many theories espoused as to the best way to manage and lead people.

Leadership, and therefore effective management, involves behavior—your behavior and the behavior of the individual or group that you are attempting to influence. Understanding what motivates people, predicting how they will respond to your leadership attempts, and directing their behavior are all necessary for effective leadership. You must be willing to accept the responsibility for influencing the behavior of others if you are to be successful in accomplishing tasks and reaching goals.

There are two basic behaviors that you will have to demonstrate in your role as a personnel manager. The first is directive, or task-oriented, behavior where you will set the goals and objectives, plan and organize the work to be done, communicate priorities, clarify roles of the workers, and constantly show and tell the worker how to do the job. The second behavior you will need is supportive, or relationship-oriented, during which you will listen to the problems of the worker that you are managing. You will praise, encourage, reassure, ask for suggestions, and communicate to the worker the hospital's plans and goals.

How you communicate these behaviors and how much emphasis you place on each will be your management style. You may use primarily directive behavior and be what is commonly know as an authoritarian or autocratic leader. If your management style uses primarily the supportive behavior, you will be known as a participative or democratic leader. These two styles of leadership are also known as the Theory X and Theory Y management styles, first popularized by Douglas McGregor in the early 1960s.[4] Theory X assumes that people prefer to be directed; are not interested in assuming responsibility; and are motivated primarily by money, fringe benefits, and the threat of punishment. Theory Y believes that people are not lazy and unreliable and can be self-directed and creative at work, if properly supported and motivated.

It should be easy to see that neither of these theories is applicable in every case, and that an effective management style will need to create a balance between the amount of direction and support that you give. It is important for you to understand, however, that it will be the worker's perception of that direction and support, not yours, that will affect behavior. You may see yourself as a humanistic and caring person, but your employee considers you hard nosed and bossy. Different employees will perhaps have different perceptions and will actually need and request different levels of direction and support. You will have to know the needs of the employees that you are managing and be able to be adaptable, depending on those needs.

For a more complete study of management styles and theories, read the following books listed in Appendix A:

- Chapter one, "Leadership Makes a Difference," of McCurnin's *Veterinary Practice Management*
- *Management of Organization Behavior* by Hersey and Blanchard
- *Leadership and the One Minute Manager* by Blanchard

You will have many important tasks as an animal hospital manager, but none will have more affect on your success and effectiveness than your role as a personnel manager. Your management style and how you control your behavior to develop that style will be a major factor in the determination of that success and effectiveness.

Defining the Job and Its Requirements

We will assume that the planning process carried out by the hospital owners has determined the staffing needs. Your first and probably most important step, that is frequently bypassed, is to create complete and accurate job descriptions. You may decide to ask staff to either write the job description or aid you in the task. A job description should include the following:

- A definition of the job. What has to be done? How does the employer or employee know when the job is done?

- What special skills does the job require? Are there educational requirements? Is experience necessary? Are any personality traits a help or a hindrance?
- What are the essential duties of the job? This should be a complete list of the duties expected to be performed by the employee. Essential duties should include not only the intellect and skill functions but also the physical, stress, and time functions. If there are secondary duties that may be required under certain circumstances, these should be listed as well. For example, if the employee is expected to be able to lift a fifty-pound dog, say so in the job description.
- What are the authority boundaries of the position? Whom does this employee report to and who will determine how well the employee is functioning? How much authority is assigned to the position?[5]

The job description is used to recruit and select new employees, train new employees, review performance, and determine salary. It serves as an initial screening device for job applicants. It defines the job, tells the prospective employee what will be expected, and tells the employer what kind of employee to look for. Job descriptions should be looked at and reconsidered at least once annually or more often in the event of staff reductions or staff growth. Appendix B has a sample job description.

The inability to perform the essential duties would make a prospective employee unqualified for the position. In the case of an otherwise qualified person who has a disability, the employer may be required to make a reasonable accommodation for that employee which would allow the disabled person to become qualified. This subject is covered in more detail under the subject of the Americans with Disabilities Act later in this chapter.

Hiring

The process of hiring a new employee involves three basic steps: recruitment, screening, and selection. The first step is to communicate to prospective employees that there is a position available. Where and how you do this will depend to a great extent on what the position is and what the requirements for the position are as determined by the job description. For example, you would not advertise for a veterinarian or a veterinary technician in the local newspaper and you would probably not try to find a receptionist in a professional journal classified section. Some commonly used sources for recruitment include the following:

- **employment agencies**—these may be government or private and would be primarily used as a source of secretarial help or unskilled labor.
- **schools**—these may be professional or trade schools. Veterinary colleges and veterinary technician programs will have procedures for recruitment of graduates. Trade schools also will be good sources for secretarial and bookkeeping help.

- **word-of-mouth**—your present employees may know someone or a neighboring hospital may have surplus help. You also may find that a client is looking for a job and may be qualified.
- **advertising**—newspaper advertising is the most commonly used source when seeking nonprofessional employees. Your newspaper advertisement should be very specific so as to eliminate those persons who do not meet the requirements of your job description. Newspaper advertisements may carry the name and address of the prospective employer or may be a blind ad, giving only a box number or a telephone number to call. Personal preference will determine how you place your advertisement. If the position to be filled is for a professional employee, you will want to place an advertisement in the appropriate professional journal.

The next step is to screen the candidates who have applied for the job. First, eliminate any candidates who do not meet the requirements as stated in the job description. Then you need to determine which of the remaining candidates is the best qualified. You can do this by any one or a combination of the following:

Letter of Qualification

Ask the candidate to send you a letter stating qualifications for the position and reasons for wanting the job. This could be done at the outset by a blind ad or could be a request after the prospective employee had responded to some other device. This is a particularly effective means to determine the prospective employee's writing skills and would be valuable if writing was an important duty in the position.

Resumé

Depending on the position, you may ask for a resumé. Resumés would be most valuable for professional or technical positions where prior education or experience is required or desired.

Telephone the Candidate

Call the candidate or ask the candidate to call you. If the position entails talking to clients or others on the telephone, as would be the case with receptionists, this is a very useful means to determine the candidate's poise as well as voice projection over the telephone.

Asking for References

Ask for references, particularly from former employers. If the prospective employee will be responsible for handling money, a financial reference is important.

The Interview

Interview the candidates that you have determined are the best. Interviews should be scheduled and should be conducted in quiet surroundings. The candidate should fill out an approved, legal application form (see Appendix B). If the position requires writing or filing, some type of spelling and grammar test should be administered (sample test in Appendix B). You also can give a typing test or a computer test if the job requires either skill. The interview should be a relaxed exchange of dialogue, with the candidate doing most of the talking. You should give a brief summary of the position and read with the candidate the job description. Then you should ask questions such as

- "Tell me about yourself." This answer will identify likes, dislikes, and prejudices.
- "What jobs have you done?" This answer will help to identify skills.
- "What attracted you to this position?" This answer will help to determine interest in the position.
- "Have you ever been discharged from a previous position?" This will help determine the reliability of the candidate.
- "How does this position fit into your long-range goals?" This should tell you about motivation.
- "Why are you leaving your present position?" This answer may reflect the suitability of the candidate.

If the position involves handling animals, it would be a good idea to discuss the candidate's fitness, both physically and emotionally, particularly with reference to euthanasia and pain on the part of the animal. You should do this by addressing the essential functions and ask the prospective employee about performing them. If the candidate establishes the existence of a disability that could prevent fulfilling the essential duties, it will be the duty of the employer, together with the candidate, to determine if the duties could be performed by providing a reasonable accommodation.

You may want to consider personality profile testing at this point. These tests, such as the Myers Briggs Type indicator (MBTI), are designed to determine which personalities might be compatible working with each other and what traits an individual possesses that would best meet the expectations of the employer. If this type of test is used prior to employment, it must be given to all candidates. Any trait or condition that could be identified by the personality tests that could be considered a disability or caused by a disability should not be used as a reason not to employ the individual. Personality tests could be more valuable to use after employment to determine which staff members would perform better in certain positions or working with certain employees. Additional information on personality testing appears in Appendix A.

Salary should be discussed frankly with a specific hourly or weekly salary offered. In addition, all benefits should be specified.[6]

Application and Interview Checklist

The guidelines shown in Table 2.1 should be considered as to what is lawful and unlawful with regard to questions that can be asked of a prospective employee on an application form or during an interview.[7]

The interviewer should have a form (see Appendix B) and should make notes during the interview. The interviewer should pay attention to the candidate's appearance, diction, use of grammar, and personality. If several candidates are to be interviewed, follow the same format as closely as possible so that you can compare the candidates.

SUBJECT	LAWFUL	UNLAWFUL
Age	Are you 18 years of age or older? If not, state your age. Do you have a work permit?	How old are you? What is your date of birth? What are the ages of your children?
Arrest record	Have you ever been convicted of a crime? If yes, give details.	Have you ever been arrested?
Marital status	None	Do you wish to be addressed as Miss? Mrs.? Ms.? Are you married? Single? Divorced? Separated? Any information about one's spouse.
Disability	None	Do you have a disability? Have you ever been treated for any of the following diseases ...? Do you have now or have you ever had a problem with alcohol or drugs?
National origin	None	Inquiry into the applicants lineage, ancestry, national origin, descent, parentage or nationality. Nationality of applicants parents.
Race or color	None	Complexion or skin coloring.
Sex	None	
Address or duration of residence	Applicant's place of residence. How long a resident of this state or city?	
Bitrhplace	None	Requirement that applicant submit birth certificate, naturalization or baptismal record.

Table 2.1 Lawful and unlawful interview questions (part 1).

Citizenship	Are you a citizen of the United States? If not a citizen of the United States, do you intend to become a citizen of the United States? If you are not a citizen, have you the legal right to remain permanently in the United States? Do you intend to remain in the United States?	Of what country are you a citizan? Whether the applicant is a naturalized or non-native-born citizen: the date when the applicant acquired citizenship. Requirement that the applicant produce naturalization papers or first papers. Whether applicant's parents are naturalized or native-born citizens of the United States; the date when parents acquired citizenship.
Driver's license	Do you possess a valid driver's license?	Requirement that the driver produce a driver's license.
Education	Inquire into the applicant's academic, vocational, or professional education and the public and private schools attended.	
Experience	Inquiry into work experience.	
Military experience	Inquiry into applicant's experience in the Armed Forces of the United States or the State Militia.	Inquiry into the applicants military experience other than the Armed Forces of the United States or the State Militia. Did you receive a discharge from the military in other than honorable circumstances?
Organizations	Inquiry into applicant's membership in organizations which the applicant considers relevant to his or her ability to perform the job.	List all clubs, societies and lodges to which you belong.
Photograph	None	Requirement or option that applicant attach photograph to employment form at any time *before* hiring

Table 2.1 Lawful and unlawful interview questions (part 2).

Tour of the Facility

After the interview is completed, give the candidate a tour of the hospital, introducing present employees and pointing out phases of the position. Remember that your best candidates can find many jobs. If they couldn't, they wouldn't be your best candidates. You may have to sell that candidate on coming to work for you. A pleasant experience during the interview, along with the perception of a nice place to work with happy coworkers, will go a long way.

Concluding the Interview

At the conclusion of the interview or tour, give the candidate a specific date when you will know the results of your hiring process. If it is obvious that the candidate does not have the necessary job requirements, you may want to say so at this time, rather than call later. You should never, however, hire a candidate until you have completed all of the interviews.

Making the Decision

The last step in the hiring process is the selection of the best candidate for the position. You should have the following information on each candidate: a completed application form, names of references, an interview form filled out by the interviewer, and other materials such as spelling tests.

Certainly for any of the candidates that you would consider hiring, you should contact the references. When calling references, have a form available (see Appendix B) that will guide you in your questions. If the reference is a former employer, you should ask the circumstances of the candidate leaving and whether the former employer would hire the candidate back if a position were available.

After you have completed the entire process and have made your decision, you should rank the candidates from the best on down. At the appointed time, call your first place candidate and offer the position before you make any other calls. You may find that the person you have selected will want to negotiate the salary that you have offered or some other part of the employment package. You should be prepared to make a counteroffer or state that you will call back after consultation with the hospital owners. Never call your next choices to inform them that they were not successful until you have hired someone. It is always possible that the person you choose will not want the position or may have accepted another.

After you have an acceptance to your job offer, you should then call the other top candidates and inform them that the position has been filled. It may be a good idea to ask those acceptable candidates whom you do not hire if they would be interested if another position were to become available. If so, keep those files for up to two years and you could very well eliminate this whole process the next time you need a new employee. Before making such an offer, however, ask your legal counsel if there could be any possible consequences that could result in legal claims against the hospital.

Training

Your hospital now has a new employee who has reported to work at the agreed upon time. What happens next? Too many times, the answer to that question is nothing. Providing new employees with proper training and proper information is essential in the development of a good working relationship. The first step on your part will be to assign the task of training the new employee to the proper person or persons. If this is a new position, you as the manager are most likely the appropriate person to do the training. If the new staff member is replacing someone who is either assuming a new position or leaving, then the person being replaced may be the appropriate person unless this person is a disgruntled employee. **NEVER** ask an employee whom you are firing or who has done an unsatisfactory job to train a new employee. You will only get another unsatisfactory performance.

The First Day

You as the manager/trainer should be sure to be at the hospital when the new employee arrives for the first day. Your new staff member should be shown where to leave coats, lunches, handbags, etc. If uniforms are to be provided, and this has not been arranged previously, provisions for this should be made. The new staff member then should be introduced to all staff members in the hospital. You should be sure to arrange for an introduction to all staff members who are not there as soon as possible.

The manager and the new employee should then go to a quiet area of the hospital where they should carefully, once again, study the job description. If the employee has been hired for a trial period, it should be made clear what the process will be at the end of that period to determine continued employment. The employer and employee should both be satisfied. The new staff member should be asked to read the hospital policies and procedures manual. The contents of this manual will be discussed later in this chapter.

Salary, benefits, general organization of the practice, management goals and philosophy, and other pertinent information should be provided in writing and discussed. The new staff member should be encouraged to ask questions, and both parties should be satisfied that all hospital policies and procedures are understood before this phase of the training is completed. Now is the time to have the new employee complete the necessary personnel forms that will include the I-9 Employment Eligibility Verification form and the W4 Withholding form for the Internal Revenue Service. Copies of these forms are in Appendix B.

On-the-Job Training

The next part of the training will be the actual on-the-job portion. This should be conducted by the individual with the highest level of knowledge of the position. The trainer should first find out what the new employee already knows about the position and what skills the new employee has that can be used. There should be at least a day or two of telling, showing, and illustrating, which will be primarily observation on the part of the new staff member. The trainer should stress key points, instruct clearly and completely, and be sure not to attempt to teach more than can be mastered in the time allowed. Do not ask your new employee to take primary responsibility for the position until the employee has been shown how to handle that responsibility. The amount of training necessary for a new employee to become effective on the job will vary tremendously from individual to individual and from position to position. As manager, you should be sure that your new staff member is capable and comfortable with the task before you turn the new employee loose. You can best make this determination by testing. When the employee does go it alone, be sure to discuss, at least once a day, how the employee feels about the progress. Encourage the employee to ask questions, and make sure that the employee knows who to go to for help.

The on-the-job training can be aided and assisted by a visual presentation using photographs or slides made by your hospital staff for the purpose of training new staff members. These can be particularly helpful in pointing out situations that do not occur frequently. There also are prepared visual presentations made for this purpose and marketed by veterinary organizations and others in the business of training. Several of these sources are identified in Appendix A. Journals or magazines that feature articles pertinent to the new employee's position also are helpful as are continuing education meetings at local community colleges, veterinary association meetings, etc.

At the appropriate time, when the new staff member appears to be comfortable with the position, it is a good idea to cross-train with other staff members. Cross-training means that more than one staff member knows how to do a particular job in case of sickness, vacation, or emergency.

Concluding the Training

There should be a prearranged time when the formal training will be concluded. At this time the new employee's performance should be reviewed. If the review is not satisfactory, the employment of the individual should not be continued. It would be hoped that sufficient warning had been given so that this occurrence would not come as a surprise to the employee. You should be sure that you and your staff have given enough time and proper training to be able to sufficiently evaluate the employee's performance. If you are still dissatisfied, do not hesitate to end the relationship.

Performance Evaluation

The evaluation process provides the hospital manager with the tools necessary for measuring and changing the performance of employees.[9] It also gives the employee the opportunity to find out how satisfied the employers are with the performance. This should be a major part of a performance evaluation but is frequently not communicated to the employee. Performance evaluations should be done at the end of the trial employment period or no more than 90 days after hiring a new staff member, and at least once a year thereafter.

The performance evaluations should not be associated with salary review except in the case of the new employee in a trial period who is to receive a salary increase at the end of a satisfactory trial period. Associating performance evaluation with salary review can only diminish or deteriorate the value of the performance review.[10]

Before the Evaluation

Prior to the actual employee evaluation, the employee's manager should go through a similar evaluation, usually done by the hospital owner. This is necessary to give the manager perspective and control of the task of evaluating other staff members. It also establishes the hierarchy of responsibility within the hospital. To do the actual evaluation, you should use some type of form (see samples in Appendix B). The form also should be given to the staff member to fill out as a self-evaluation. The manager should carefully complete the same form on the employee to be evaluated.

The Evaluation Meeting

At the evaluation, which will be a face-to-face meeting of the manager and employee in a quiet, relaxed, and uninterrupted setting, the manager and employee should compare evaluations. The manager should show and read the manager's evaluation of the employee to the employee, pointing out areas of agreement in the employee's self-evaluation. If there are areas of major concern about the employee's performance, the manager should be sure to have specifics and documentation for the concerns. The employee's performance should be compared to the job description. The employee should not be faulted for not performing tasks not in the job description. The employee should be asked for comments and if there is agreement or disagreement with the evaluation and why. The manager should offer suggestions as to how the employee can improve and correct problem areas and offer praise for areas in which the employee's performance exceeds expectations. The employee should be allowed to ask questions and give comments on working conditions, chances for advancement, and overall job satisfaction.

The evaluation procedure is too often not done in many businesses, including animal hospitals. It is often perceived by both the manager and the employee as placing the two of them in an adversarial situation. In reality, nothing could be further from the truth. A properly executed performance evaluation can have a positive effect on a business and the human relations within the management of that business. The key will be whether or not the manager has, and demonstrates, that most important skill of management—the ability to communicate.

Compensation Methods and Discussion

Presumably in their planning function, the hospital owners have included a budget with an amount for salaries and benefits. As the manager, you may be given salary ranges for hiring employees for specific positions, or you may be given a salary budget with the authority to allocate salaries at your discretion. In some cases, you may have no authority other than that of a recommendation. You may use written contracts in all cases or perhaps only in select cases, or all employees might be hired under terms of verbal contracts. In any case, it will be your responsibility to communicate salaries and other forms of compensation to employees. A common mistake on the part of employees is to consider only the hourly or weekly salary as the total compensation. Compensation of employees includes all or most of the following, and it is your job to communicate this information.

- hourly or weekly salary
- employer's portion of Social Security (FICA) payment
- employer's taxes on unemployment, disability, and workers' compensation
- applicable local, state, or provincial taxes
- sick pay and personal days off with pay
- vacation and paid holidays
- health insurance and major medical plans
- pension and profit sharing plans
- life insurance
- uniform allowance
- professional dues and subscriptions
- continuing education payment or assistance
- veterinary care for pets
- bonding and malpractice insurance where applicable

The elements of compensation other than salary often add from 25 to 30 percent to the costs of hiring an employee. It is important that this is well communicated and understood. You should do so at the time of the initial interview with the prospective employee, then repeat the information on the first day of employment and constantly thereafter by means of the hospital policies and procedures manual. And always include this information at the time of salary review.

A salary review should be done annually and consistently for each employee. The options that you or the owners have are to give no salary increases to anyone, to give increases to selected employees, or to give a percentage or set amount increase to everyone.

Which choice is used will be decided by the constraints of the hospital budget and the philosophy of the management. No increase will certainly create disgruntled employees who may feel they have actually lost buying power because of inflation. Increases to selected employees with none to others has the obvious problems associated with it but may be used as a motivational device. The decision may be to increase all employees a certain amount which can either be a percentage of present salary or a set amount per hour or week. If you feel that certain employees deserve a higher increase than others, you may add performance increases or bonuses as well. The basic difference between an increase and a bonus is that an increase is permanent and a bonus is a one-time payment that should not be expected to be repeated.

In addition, some hospitals may decide to give bonuses or a percentage of sales to employees as incentives for sales of certain products such as dog foods or insecticides. There are other innovative ways that employees can be compensated for efforts on behalf of your hospital. Ethical considerations should dictate that nonveterinary employees should never be paid for recommending or inducing clients to purchase medical goods or services.[12] The one constant, however, will be the necessity to communicate the methods of compensation to the employees. Handing them a weekly paycheck alone is not enough.

Termination of Employment

In most states in the United States, employment is considered to be "at will." Employment "at will" means that unless a specific provision in an employment contract stated an agreed-upon duration of employment, employees may quit and employers may terminate as a matter of their own preference. There are many exceptions. Federal statutes, organized labor and labor contracts have significantly reduced the scope of the "at will" doctrine of employment. Express exceptions to "at will" employment would include the following:

- Collective bargaining agreements.
- Specific contracts which indicate a definite period of employment.
- The Civil Rights Act prohibits dismissals based on race, sex, color, creed, or national origin.
- The Age Discrimination Act prohibits dismissals based on age if over 40 years old.
- The Pregnancy Discrimination Act prohibits dismissal because of pregnancy.
- The Occupational Safety and Health Act prohibits dismissals because employees refuse to work in a workplace that they consider unsafe or if they have exercised their rights under the Act.
- The Bankruptcy Reform Act prohibits dismissal of an employee because he or she has filed for bankruptcy.
- Federal law prohibits dismissal of an employee because of his or her service on a federal jury.

Employers may also be accused of wrongful discharge of an employee for reasons of public policy (i.e., refusing to commit perjury, refusal to price fix or whistle blowing), implied contract rights (i.e., oral contract or a statement in an employee handbook implying a term of employment), or implied covenant of good faith and fair dealing (i.e., accusal of not acting in good faith).[11]

The catalyst for a wrongful discharge claim often can be an inappropriately handled notice of termination—a notice that is poorly timed, poorly stated, and/or too publicly handled. A discharged employee who feels that he or she has been humiliated is much more likely to sue. In most instances, the decision to terminate employment may not be as critically important as how that decision is carried out.

Firing an Employee

The one thing you hope you will never have to do is fire an employee. However, it may be necessary under circumstances such as the following:

- unsatisfactory performance of duties;
- excessive tardiness and absenteeism;
- dishonest or unethical behavior in the performance of duties;
- criminal activity within the hospital (such as stealing) or outside the hospital (such as drug abuse), either of which has been substantiated by a criminal investigation;
- elimination of the position by a management decision.

Having considered everything in the preceding paragraph about the exceptions to at-will employment and having carefully documented the reasons for termination of the employee, the following rules should be considered and used:

- Don't spend your time and energy trying to avoid it. Delays between the employee action and the discipline on your part will be viewed as indecisiveness by the other employees and will threaten your ability to manage effectively.
- Be sure that the decision to fire was preceded by a series of clear, understood, and documented discussions with the employee. If you are firing an employee for unsatisfactory performance of duties, the first time that the employee finds out that you are dissatisfied should not be at the firing.
- Don't fire an employee in haste when you are angry at the time of a transgression.
- Do it in private, preferably at the end of the day, so that the fired employee will not have to encounter other employees after the firing.
- Be honest, control emotions, and do the firing with dignity.

- Unless the firing is due to a reason unrelated to the employee's performance of duties, it is best not to let the employee work after the firing. Concern for getting the job done and your need for a worker until you can replace the fired employee may encourage this decision. However, this situation could have a very disconcerting affect on the rest of your staff.
- At the time of the firing, have all earned money ready to give to the fired employee, including earned vacation time and back salary. Ask the dismissed employee to sign a release foregoing his or her right to sue over the dismissal. Depending on the circumstances, you may want to provide severance pay as a means to obtain this release.
- If you have provided health care benefits, you may want to offer to continue them, at the individual's expense, for a period of time. The Consolidated Omnibus Budget Reconciliation Act of 1986 (COBRA) allows for the extension of group insurance coverage to employees and their dependents on a self-pay basis. COBRA requires employers to cover former employees whose medical condition would prevent them from immediately getting coverage under a new employer plan.
- Ask the fired employee to remove personal property from the hospital and to return keys or any other hospital property. Try to eliminate any reason for the employee to return to the hospital. In some cases, you may want to change the locks on the hospital doors.
- Depending on the circumstances of the firing, you may or may not be willing to give the employee a reference for another job. You should discuss your intentions in this regard with the fired employee.
- Document the firing, the circumstances preceding it, and the reaction of the fired employee in writing, and place it in the employee's personnel file. If you are accused of wrongful discharge, proper and complete documentation of the entire process will be absolutely necessary. If you have any questions as to whether or not you may have such a problem, it would be wise to discuss the situation with your attorney *before* you decide to fire the employee.[13]

Your ability to fire will be as important as your ability to hire. If you have an employee who is not performing or is the source of a problem, the sooner you remove that employee, the better your hospital will be.

Personnel Records

Each employee who works for your hospital should have a separate file in which all materials related to employment are stored. These files should be kept in a locked, secure cabinet that is accessible only to management. An individual employee should be able to see his or her file, but only by request and in the presence of management. A personnel record should contain the following:

- original application, records of contacts with references, and resumé, if required;
- an employee record form (sample in Appendix B) that shows date of hire, original salary, record of raises, and other employment history;
- performance evaluations;
- attendance and vacation records (samples in Appendix B);
- a written record of reprimands or other discussions related to performance of duties;
- records of benefits such as medical payments received;
- records and documentation of any injuries suffered while working and any resulting claims;
- a well-documented record of firing (if applicable).

If the employee decides to leave, there should be an exit interview that should be a frank exchange of the reasons for leaving and the employee's job satisfaction. This exit interview also should be documented and made a permanent part of the employee's file.

The period of time that you should keep a personnel file after an employee leaves is a matter that you should discuss with your accountant or attorney. In no case should a file be kept less than five years.

Consult the local office of the United States Department of Labor and any state or provincial labor authorities for rules and regulations enforced in your state or province that control such things as hiring of minors, special considerations for female workers, civil rights, rights of disabled workers, notices that should be on display for employees, minimum wages and rules pertaining to overtime, and recording of working hours as well as how long records are to be kept.

Time records are important to answer inquiries that may be presented to you by government authorities. A time clock is an efficient and generally acceptable way to keep time records and should be considered by your hospital if one is not currently in use.

Employment Laws

Every aspect of personnel management is affected and controlled by some form of law, and new laws are created frequently. The following are most of the federal laws of the United States that must be considered with regard to personnel management.[14] In addition, most states have companion laws that supplement, change the requirements of, or supersede the federal laws. Many states also have additional laws pertaining to personnel management. Canadian readers should check with their provincial registrar for applicable laws.

Immigration Control

The Immigration Reform and Control Act affects all employers. It contains several provisions which require employers to institute procedures for verifying that a job applicant is authorized to be employed in the United States. All employers must verify that every new hire is either a U.S. citizen or is authorized to work in this country. The act also requires employers to state on Immigration and Naturalization Form I-9 (a copy is in Appendix B) that they have examined the necessary documents that show that the individual is not an unauthorized alien. The new hire must also attest on the verification form that he or she qualifies for employment. The verification forms must be retained for three years from the date of hire or one year from the date of termination, whichever is longer.

The Fair Labor Standards Act

The Fair Labor Standards Act (FLSA) sets basic minimum wage and overtime pay standards and regulates the employment of minors. Congress changes the minimum wage frequently, and some states have laws that supersede the federal minimum wage. The hospital manager should ascertain what the current minimum wage is for the appropriate state. The work week—seven consecutive, regular recurring, 24-hour periods of 168 hours—is the unit of time used for determining compliance with the minimum wage. The overtime pay premium (one and one-half times the regular rate) applies to all hours worked above forty in a workweek. The employer is required to have posted, in an obvious location, the standard workplace poster on the federal minimum wage.

In circumstances where an employee must wear a uniform, the financial burden of furnishing and maintaining (including laundry and repair) the uniform may not be imposed on the employee if the resulting wage would be below minimum wage or overtime compensation required by the FLSA.

The FLSA provides for an exemption from both the minimum wage and overtime pay provisions for employees engaged in an executive, administrative or professional capacity. In the case of the professional employee, the individual's primary duty must be in work requiring knowledge of advanced type of science or learning, original work in an artistic field or teaching.

Employers are required to keep records on wages, hours, and other items for three years. Records required for exempt employees differ from those for non-exempt employees, and special information is required about employees working under uncommon pay arrangements.

The hospital manager should be aware of the many other requirements of the FLSA. These include the minimum wage, overtime pay, and other items such as commission pay, holidays, bonuses, trainees, learners and handicapped workers, part-time employees, and child labor. Additional information should be requested from the U.S Department of Labor.

Employees/Independent Contractors

Whether an individual is classified as an employee or an independent contractor has far-reaching consequences when determining a business's responsibility for the individual under the Fair Labor Standards Act; to determine liability under the Federal Insurance Contribution Act (FICA) and the Federal Unemployment Tax Act (FUTA); determining income tax withholding responsibilities and liability for providing benefits to an individual under evolving sections of the Internal Revenue code. It is no easy matter to determine whether an employee is an independent contractor, and there have been many court cases disputing this issue over the years. The Internal Revenue Service uses a set of 20 Common Law Factors to determine if an employer-employee relationship exists. These Common Law Factors are listed in Figure 2.1. Under the common law test, an individual generally is an employee if the person for whom the individual performs service has the right to control and direct that individual, both as to the details and the means by which the result of that service is to be accomplished.

Civil Rights

With the historic passage of the Civil Rights Act of 1964, it became the law of the land to bring about equal opportunity for all in the crucial area of employment rights. Discrimination under this act was defined as the failure or refusal to hire, to discharge, or to discriminate against any individual with respect to compensation, terms, conditions, or privileges of employment because of such individual's race, color, religion, sex, or national origin. The Equal Employment Opportunity Commission (EEOC) was created to enforce this anti-discrimination law. Although all businesses, regardless of size, are expected to not discriminate, only those businesses with 15 or more employees come under the jurisdiction of the EEOC with regard to the Civil Rights Act. Every employer must post an official Equal Employment Opportunity poster in a conspicuous location frequented by employees.

Sexual Harassment

Although sexual discrimination and sexual harassment were covered by the 1964 Civil Rights Act, sexual harassment claims have risen dramatically since 1985. The EEOC has issued guidelines which define two types of sexual harassment: "quid pro quo" and "environmental." The former includes unwelcome sexual conduct when submission to or rejection of such conduct by an individual is used as the basis of employment decisions affecting the individual. The latter includes unwelcome sexual conduct that unreasonably interferes with the individual's job performance or creates an "intimidating, hostile, or offensive working environment," even if it leads to no tangible or economic job consequence. Sexist jokes, nude pictures displayed or in a magazine kept out in the open, touching after being requested not to do so, or criticism with sexist connotations could all be

- Is the individual providing services required to comply with the instructions concerning when, where, and how the work is to be done?
- Is the individual provided with training to enable him or her to perform a job in a particular manner?
- Are the services performed by the indiviaul integrated into the business's operations?
- Must the services be rendered personally?
- Does the business hire, supervise, or pay assistants to help the individual performing the services under contract?
- Is the relationship between the individual and the person for whom he or she performs services a continuing relationship?
- Who sets the hours of work?
- Is the individual required to devote full time to the person for whom he or she performs services?
- Does the individual perform work on another's business premises?
- Who directs the order or sequence on which the work must be done?
- Are regular oral or written reports required?
- What is the method of payment—hourly, weekly, commission, or by the job?
- Are business or travel expenses reimbursed?
- Who furnishes tools and materials necessary for the provision of services?
- Can the individual providing services realize a profit or loss?
- Can the individual providing services work for a number of firms at the same time?
- Does the individual make his or her services available to the general public?
- Is the individual providing services subject to dismissal for reasons other than nonperformance of contract specifications?
- Can the individual providing services terminate his or her relationship at any time without incuring liability for failure to complete a job?

Figure 2.1 I.R.S. Common Law Factors for determining independent contractor status considered sexual harassment. There should be a policy on sexual harassment either posted on a bulletin board or in the hospital policy manual. A sample is included in Appendix B.

Pregnancy Discrimination

The Pregnancy Discrimination Act of 1978 makes it clear that discrimination on the basis of pregnancy, childbirth, or related medical conditions constitutes unlawful sex discrimination under the Civil Rights Act. The basic principle of the act is that women affected by pregnancy and related conditions must be treated the same as other applicants and employees on the basis of their ability or inability to work.

Other EEOC Guidelines

There are also EEOC guidelines regarding discrimination related to religion, national origin, and affirmative action.

The Americans with Disabilities Act

In 1990, Congress passed the Americans with Disabilities Act (ADA) which brings individuals with disabilities under the protection of the Civil Rights Act. Disability means a physical or mental impairment that substantially limits one or more of the major life functions of an individual. The law covers employers who have 15 or more employees (including part-time) for each working day in each of 20 or more calendar weeks in the current or preceding year. Title One of the ADA prohibits employers covered under the act from discriminating against any qualified individual with a disability with respect to practically every aspect of the employment relationship. This includes job application procedures, hiring, advancement, discipline, discharge, compensation, job training, leave, benefits, and all other terms, conditions, and privileges of employment. The term *qualified person with a disability* is defined as an individual "who satisfies the requisite skill experience, education, and other job-related requirements of the position such individual holds or desires, and who, with or without the assistance of a reasonable accommodation, can perform the *essential functions* of such position."

Written job descriptions that specify essential tasks of the position that are prepared before advertising and interviewing are very important. This job description or job task list shall be considered evidence of the essential functions of the job. It should include not only the intellectual and skill functions but also the physical, time, and stress functions. If the job requires that the individual be able to lift a 50-pound dog or bag of dog food, say so in the job description.

If an individual, except for limitations caused by a disability, is qualified to perform the essential functions of a job, the employer must consider whether or not the individual could perform these functions with the assistance of a *reasonable accommodation.* A reasonable accommodation is a modification or adjustment to a job or the work environment that enables a qualified applicant or an employee with a disability to participate in the application process or to perform the job. The employer is expected to make reasonable accommodations if, with that accommodation, the individual with the disability can perform the essential functions of the position that the individual holds or has applied to hold. A reasonable accommodation must be made unless the accommodation would impose an undue hardship on the operation of the business. Reasonable accommodations would include

- job restructuring,
- making work and non-work areas accessible and usable,
- part-time or modified work schedules,
- adjustments and modifications to pre-employment exams and training programs,
- reassignment to vacant positions,
- providing accommodation aids such as telephone head sets, electronic visual aids, magnifiers, and telephone amplifiers,
- lowering or raising desks,
- providing assistants such as interpreters, and
- providing reserved parking places.

The term *undue hardship* means significant difficulty, disruption of business, or expense incurred by the covered entity. It will be covered on a case-by-case basis that will take into consideration the nature and cost of the accommodation as well as the size and the financial resources of the business. Undue hardship must be proven by the business.

Under the ADA, an employer may not ask about the existence, nature, or severity of a disability and may not conduct medical examinations until after it makes a conditional job offer to the applicant. Medical examinations can be required after a conditional job offer is made, but an exam must be required in all such cases. The physician performing the examination should have a copy of the job description and can be asked if, in their opinion, the prospective employee is qualified. Employers may ask, at the pre-offer stage, about an applicant's ability to perform specific job-related functions, i.e., the essential functions as listed in the job description.

An employer may also ask other questions that are not disability-related and may require examinations that are not medical. Such examinations could include physical and intellectual capacity examinations (spelling, typing, or grammar tests) before the job is offered but only if all applicants are given the same test and if a direct tie between the test and the essential functions of the job is shown.

The ADA also protects existing employees from discrimination because of a disability that may occur during employment or if the employer becomes covered during that employee's tenure.

There is a list of information sources pertaining to the ADA in Appendix B. It is extremely important for the hospital manager to have complete knowledge of the hospital's responsibilities regarding its employees.

Family and Medical Leave

The Family and Medical Leave Act became effective August 5, 1993, and covers employers with 50 or more employees for each working day during 20 or more calendar weeks in all business locations located within a 75-mile radius. An eligible employee will be entitled to a total of 12 work weeks of unpaid leave during any 12-month period for one of the following reasons:

- Birth of a child of the employee in order to care for the child.
- Placement of a child with the employee for adoption or foster care.
- Care for a spouse, child, or parent of the employee if such relative has a serious health problem.
- Serious health condition that makes the employee unable to perform the functions of the position that they hold.

Except for highly compensated employees, any eligible employee who takes the leave will be entitled, on return from such leave, to be restored by the employer to the position held by the employee before leave commenced, or to an equivalent position.

Age Discrimination

In 1967, Congress passed the Age Discrimination in Employment Act (ADEA) to prohibit discrimination in employment because of age in such matters as hiring, job retention, compensation and other terms, conditions, and privileges of employment. The ADEA prohibits most employers from discrimination in employment practices against persons over 40 on the basis of their age.

Occupational Safety and Health

In 1970, Congress passed legislation establishing the Occupational Safety and Health Administration (OSHA) within the Department of Labor. OSHA requires that all employers, regardless of the number of employees, shall furnish a place of employment which is free from recognized hazards that are causing or are likely to cause death or serious physical harm to their employees. OSHA is authorized to issue workplace safety standards which are legally enforceable. Such standards include limitations on worker exposure to hazardous chemicals and maximum workplace noise levels. OSHA has the authority to conduct workplace inspections and impose substantial citations and penalties for workplace conditions which violate OSHA regulations. No other federal law or agency brings as much concern to the animal hospital owner and manager as does OSHA. Given the broad scope of the law and the fact that it requires employers to undertake certain affirmative action to educate and train workers, it is important that every employer become familiar with the basic law. Programs such as the "OSHA Compliance Guide for Veterinary Practices" and the "Hazardous Materials Training Program," both available from AAHA, must be a part of the hospital manager's tools for the proper management of the hospital. Both resources include the OSHA-required "Job Safety and Health" poster that must be posted in a conspicuous location frequented by employees.

Workers' Compensation

The basic tenet of workers' compensation laws is that employers are to provide compensation in the form of wage replacement and the cost of all reasonable and necessary hospital, surgical, and medical expenses for all accidental injuries, illnesses, or death arising out of and in the course of employment. Each of the 50 states has its own workers' compensation laws, and virtually every employer is covered by these laws. Depending on the state, employers are required to obtain insurance or prove financial ability to carry their own risk. The hospital managers should be aware of the laws in their state.

Unemployment Insurance

Unemployment insurance is a national social insurance program whose major objective is to provide unemployed workers the means of getting through a temporary period of involuntary unemployment. Virtually all employers are covered, and the program is financed almost entirely from employer taxes. The employer pays both a state and a federal tax. All claimants, in order to qualify for benefits, must be able and available for suitable work. All states disqualify persons who voluntarily quit without good cause, are discharged for misconduct, or refuse an offer of suitable work.

Pensions

The Employee Retirement Income Security Act (ERISA) does not require that employees be covered by a pension plan, but once they are, the ERISA provides safeguards for the employees' interests in the plan. To protect the rights of participants, the ERISA imposes certain plan requirements. Any employer who provides a pension plan for their employees must be knowledgeable of the provisions of the ERISA.

Polygraph Protection

The Employee Polygraph Protection Act prohibits employers from directly or indirectly requiring, suggesting, or causing any employee or prospective employee to take or submit to any lie detector test. Furthermore, an employer may not discharge, discipline, discriminate against in any way, deny employment or promotion to, or threaten to take any action against any employee or prospective employee who refuses, declines, or fails to take or submit to any lie detector test or on the basis of any lie detector test results. Every employer, regardless of the number of employees, must post and maintain a Department of Labor poster on polygraph protection in a conspicuous location frequented by employees.

Required Reports

Every hospital manager must be aware of all laws pertaining to personnel as well as the reports required to satisfy the requirements of the law.

Staff Meetings

Most animal hospitals have several employees and most will have schedules that mean all employees are never on the premises at the same time. How then will you, the manager, communicate to all employees new information about pricing, techniques, vaccination procedures that the doctors have decided to recommend, or seasonal marketing programs to increase the hospital's business? A most appropriate means is the staff meeting. A staff meeting should be a time when as many hospital employees as possible meet for the express purposes of exchanging information and becoming educated to better perform duties. Here are some ideas to help you more effectively hold staff meetings to accomplish these purposes.

- Hold meetings regularly at least once a month. Lunch is the best time and meetings are best held away from the practice. Close the hospital for the period or leave one employee to cover. This role should be rotated among employees.
- The hospital should pay for the lunch as well as pay the employee for the time spent. Employees not normally working at that time should be encouraged to attend and they should be paid for the time as well.
- It is critical that each meeting have an agenda. You might consider rotating the responsibility of determining the agenda and organizing the meeting among staff members. There must be a time limit.
- At every meeting the agenda should include introduction of new staff members, any new office procedures, and an opportunity for each staff member to voice any concerns.
- Seasonal topics, such as heartworm, fleas, and ticks, should be discussed by knowledgeable staff members.
- Consideration should be given to inviting guests such as representatives of pharmaceutical companies or other suppliers to give presentations to increase the staff's knowledge.

- **A history of the hospital**
- **An organization chart, the hospital's purposes and goals, and the owner's philosophies**
- **Job descriptions for all positions**
- **What the employee needs to know**
  a. dress code
  b. policy on breaks, lunches, smoking, absences, tardiness, and use of telephones
  c. work scheduling policy
- **Personnel guidelines**
  a. salary and benefits, including sick leave and annual leave
  b. probationary period for new employee
  c. training program
  d. regulations on promotion
  e. evaluation process
  f. maternity leave
  g. how to air complaints
  h. disciplinary procedures
  i. jury and military leave
  j. continuing education requirements
  k. required notice for termination of employment
- **Safety procedures**
  a. building security
  b. fire evacuation
  c. reporting accidents
- **Hospital procedures**
  a. handling of money
  b. granting of credit
  c. check cashing procedure
  d. invoicing procedure
  e. telephone answering policy
  f. handling of emergencies
  g. abandoned animals
  h. recommended vaccination procedures
  i. prescription refill procedure
  j. handling abusing or criminal activity

Figure 2.2 Suggestions for a Policies and Procedures Manual

- Minutes of the meeting should be kept and distributed to those in attendance as well as to those unable to attend.
- A bulletin board or suggestion box should be available for employees to make suggestions for the agenda or speakers for the next meeting.

Staff meetings are an excellent means to increase your ability to manage by achieving better communications with the employees. Staff meetings that are well planned result in a better educated staff who will be more effective with clients.

Hospital Policies and Procedures Manual

Every business should have a document which outlines the policies and procedures under which the business operates (see Figure 2.2). This is called a policies and procedures manual, which is a useful tool for training and communicating with your staff. Such a manual will go a long way to promote greater understanding and teamwork among your staff. These manuals should be updated when necessary and available to the employees at all times. Care must be taken in writing these manuals because they can sometimes constitute the terms of a contractual agreement even without a signed contract. Violation of the terms of the manual could be considered breach of contract on the part of the owners.[15] Clearly state in large print in front of the manual that it is not a contract. After new employees read the manual, they should be asked to sign a statement that they have read it. After many changes are made, all employees should read the changes and sign a statement. It would be wise to have the manual checked by an attorney before publishing it.

AAHA Guide to Creating an Employee Handbook

The American Animal Hospital Association has a publication entitled *Guide to Creating an Employee Handbook*. This guide, which is available from AAHA in book or computer disk form, covers many topics that should be considered in a hospital policies and procedures manual with suggested format and wording. This handbook should be considered by any hospital manager writing a new manual or revising an existing one.

Other Considerations in Personnel Management

There are many other areas that you will have to be aware of and knowledgeable in to be an effective personnel manager. Some of these are conflict resolution between staff members or between management and staff, motivation of employees, disciplinary action for employees, dealing with problem employees, and counseling employees with personal problems.[16]

This manual can in no way deal effectively with all of the many situations that you will encounter. As stated at the outset of this manual, the definition of management was in part, "accomplishing the objectives of an organization through the effective and efficient use of others." It should be obvious to you now that that is no small or simple task.

References

1. Paul Hersey and Ken Blanchard, *Management of Organizational Behavior,* Prentice Hall, fourth edition, p. 84
2. *Harvard Business Review*, Volume 66, Number 3, May-June 1988, p. 90
3. Hersey, p. 85
4. Hersey, p. 48
5. Priscilla K. Stockner, MS, DVM, MBA, *A Practice Management Manual For Veterinarians*, Stockner and Associates, Chapter 13
6. Dennis M. McCurnin, DVM, *Veterinary Practice Management*, J.B. Lippincott Co., p. 50
7. Sheldon I. London, *How to Comply With Federal Employee Laws*, London Publishing Company, New Revised Edition 1991, pg. 2
8. Stockner, Chapter 13
9. McCurnin, p. 57
10. Stockner, Chapter 13
11. London, Chapter 15
12. Jerrold Tannenbaum, MA, JD, *Veterinary Ethics*, Williams and Wilkins, p. 303
13. Stockner, Chapter 13
14. London, Chapters 2, 3, 4, 5, 7, 8 9, 11, 12
15. Tannenbaum, p. 304
16. McCurnin, p. 63-66

Chapter 3

FRONT OFFICE AND HOSPITAL PROCEDURES

Telephone Usage

Unquestionably, the telephone is the most important instrument that you have in your hospital. It is the source of nearly all of the hospital's business and the first contact that the clients have with the hospital. Uncontrolled, the telephone can be your biggest enemy and the biggest single cause of client dissatisfaction. It is very important, therefore, that the management of telephone use by the manager and the staff receives a very high priority.

Telephone Installation

It is important that there are enough telephone lines coming into the hospital. If it appears that the phones are busy most of the time, ask the telephone company to do a busy survey. They can ascertain what the use is and if a large number of your clients are getting busy signals when they call. If that is the case, your hospital should consider one or more additional incoming lines, such as "rabbit lines." These are telephone lines that are set up so if one line is busy, the incoming call will automatically connect with an unused line.

Determine your telephone usage with a survey of your own. You can keep track of both incoming and outgoing calls for a test period to determine if you can make better use of your phone lines by directing certain types of calls, such as owners checking on hospital patients, to specific time periods. Appendix C has sample telephone usage analysis sheets.

Add a telephone line that is not publicized to clients for use as an outgoing call line. This line would be for doctors and staff and would eliminate tying up incoming lines for outgoing calls.

Never have more telephone lines than the person responsible for answering them can answer. None of your clients will appreciate getting a constant busy signal but that may be preferable to getting no answer if the receptionist is unable to handle the incoming calls. If heavy incoming calls occur only at certain times, you may consider using an outside answering service to answer calls for a short period. Of course, the alternative is to add more staff to answer the telephones.

The location of the telephones is an important consideration. Telephones should be located in proximity to the appointment books. There should be telephones located in areas where doctors, technicians, the bookkeeper, and the manager can talk without excessive noise or interruption. It will be the doctors' decision as to whether or not there should be telephones installed in examination rooms.

There are many sophisticated and automated telephone instruments and services available from telephone companies and other sources which should be part of the telephone installation in most animal hospitals. Be aware, however, not to fall into a trap of becoming so automated that personal contact with the client making the incoming call is lost. Study carefully what is available, determine what will be the hospital's needs and philosophy concerning telephone service and its management, and purchase or rent only what is required.

Answering the Telephone

Who should answer the telephone? The members of your staff who answer the telephone should be carefully chosen. A pleasant, confident, and understandable voice on the other end of a telephone can be an excellent way to gain new clients and keep the old clients satisfied. When you choose your staff members whose job descriptions include answering the telephone, you should consider their ability to project the image that you desire over the telephone.

How should the phone be answered? When possible, the telephone should be answered by the third ring. The staff member should identify the hospital and themselves such as "This is the ABC animal hospital, Mary speaking, may I help you?" The personal identification is extremely important, because, after it is given, the client is speaking to a person and not a hospital. This gives the client an immediate relationship with the staff.[1]

When answering multiple lines that have hold buttons, some very simple and important rules must be made and followed. First, **NEVER** put anyone on hold before they have had a chance to identify their problem. If the problem is an emergency, it should be dealt with promptly. Second, **NEVER** leave anyone on hold for longer than 30 seconds. For new employees, you may want to place a timer near the telephone to prevent this from happening. And third, when a call is put on hold, the staff member should write down who is on hold in order to remember the name of the person on hold. The hold button on the telephone has been called "the most dangerous piece of plastic in the office."[2] If it's abused, it is a sure means to lose and dissatisfy clients.

You should also check with your telephone company and telephone equipment vendors about the availability of a telephone call sequencer which will stack calls so that the person answering the telephone knows which one should be answered next.

Establish a manual with pertinent details on how to answer the telephone, what information to get, how to record it, and other necessary information. You may wish to include in the manual answers to frequently asked questions. Develop and include in the manual a policy on how certain calls such as emergency, personal, pet health questions, progress reports, and business calls are to be handled. There are sample call-handling worksheets in Appendix C.

Develop a policy as to what to say and what not to say. Many times the same thing said in different ways will have much different meanings to the caller. Nancy Friedman, "The Telephone Doctor," in one of her videotapes on proper telephone use, talks of the "five forbidden phrases" and how to avoid them.[3] These forbidden phrases are

- "I don't know."
- "We don't do that."
- "You'll have to...."
- "Just a second."
- "No, we don't."

Friedman suggests that instead of these phrases, say

- "Let's find out."
- "Here's what you do."
- "You'll need to...."
- "That may take a few minutes."
- Any positive alternative to "no, we don't."

Emergency Telephone Service

The hospital that you are managing may have an answering service or an automatic answering machine to answer the telephone when the hospital is closed. Before a service is hired to answer the telephone, be sure that you have recommendations from other users. In addition, periodically call the hospital number and check on the responses that the hospital clients are receiving. You may not be happy. You should expect the service to render the same telephone service and courtesy that is given by the hospital staff. If that is not the case, try to improve it by speaking to the manager of the service or, if necessary, change services. Automatic answering machines are very sophisticated today. If they are used by your hospital, be sure that the message the client hears is understandable. Be sure that the caller has all of the same options as if the call were being answered by the hospital staff.

Managing the Telephone

As a manager, you have a right to expect that the staff members you are managing will follow the rules and policies developed for the functional operation of the hospital. There is no area in which this is more important than with the telephone. Develop the policies, publish them in the hospital policies and procedures manual, monitor your staff members' telephone conversations periodically, and call the hospital and pretend to be a client to find out what type of reception you would get if you were a client. When you develop client satisfaction surveys, which are discussed later, be sure to include questions about the staff's telephone answering etiquette. Your success as a manager has no greater measurement than this.

Appointment Scheduling

The difference between a controlled and efficient practice and a chaotic one lies in the execution of a smooth appointment system. The key to providing a smooth appointment system will be the appointment book and how it is used. Some practices may use a computer for appointment scheduling. The same principles should apply whether the appointment scheduling is done manually or by computer.

Appointment Book Criteria

Each hospital should develop its own schedule based on the number of doctors and the time to be allotted to each patient. An effective appointment schedule organizes appointments realistically by keeping clients from waiting but still leaves room for emergencies. It identifies special requests or circumstances and provides for efficient use of personnel and facilities by not allowing too much nonproductive time. It also shows when the doctor will be available and, in the case of a hospital with more than one doctor, when each doctor is available. The appointment book itself should be located near the telephone as well as the client reception area and should be large enough to write in. There are sample appointment schedules in Appendix C.

Making the Appointment

Get the caller's name and telephone number and the name of the patient in order to pull the record if the animal has been in before. If it is a new patient, you may want to get enough information to prepare a record card. Find out what service is being requested and approximately how much time will be required. Is the appointment for a new puppy or kitten or for a bird or exotic animal that may require more than the usual amount of time? Is there a special request for a certain doctor? Is the appointment for a technician procedure?

Appointment Problems

"No shows" are usually habitual offenders. Make a notation on the offenders' files and call them the day of their appointments as a reminder.

"Walk-ins" should never be taken before a waiting client who is scheduled for an appointment. Try not to turn them away but do not upset the appointment schedule to accommodate walk-ins. Ask them to please make an appointment before they come again.

Some people come early to their appointments. "Early birds" may have had to wait for their appointments on a previous visit. If you are getting an unusual number of established clients showing up early for their appointments, you may have an appointment scheduling problem.

Clients dropping off or picking up patients may need to talk to the doctor. These clients should be given regular appointments ahead of time or spaces should be left in the appointment schedule to accommodate them.

Review the appointment schedule at least daily. Try to correct problems before they arise. Review the scheduling format periodically and make changes as they are required. Do not learn to live with a bad system.

Reception of Clients and Patients

Without clients, the hospital that you are managing has no patients, and without patients, the hospital has no business. In most small animal practices, the clients' first contact with the practice will be with the receptionist. New clients will make some preliminary conclusions about the practice within their first two to five minutes in the reception area.[4] Greeting clients and pets by name when they enter the hospital will go a long way to make a good first impression. As clients arrive the receptionist should check the appointment list for their names. How well you have succeeded in your choice of receptionist and training of the receptionist, and how effective the materials that the hospital has provided to the reception area to communicate its services to the client will determine, to a great extent, how successful those few minutes are. In the case of a repeat client who has been to the hospital before, the client has returned because of satisfaction with the service given on previous visits. Although the first impression with a repeat client is not as important, it is no less important that this client be treated with the same courtesy and concern as the new client or the "old" client may decide to make this visit the last one.

Each new client should be asked to provide information required by the hospital to complete its records. This information should include at least the following:

- name and address
- spouse's name
- telephone numbers—home and business
- occupation
- information on all owned pets—species, breed, sex, age, neutering and vaccination history, previous medical history of significance

This registration form also may be used to gain information from the new client pertaining to how the hospital was chosen. If the hospital is computerized, there may be other information that will be requested. There are sample owner and pet registration forms in Appendix C.

The appointment schedule should eliminate most waiting time but it is unlikely that there will be none. The reception area of the hospital should maintain an atmosphere that will make this waiting as painless as possible. Here are some things that may be done to accomplish this.

- a VCR with tapes on common problems relating to the health care of animals
- a play corner for children or a fish tank
- bulletin boards with information on animal health care and community information pertaining to pets such as obedience training classes
- a bulletin board with informal pictures of clients and pets of the hospital with an open invitation for clients to add their own favorite pictures
- free coffee

The waiting area should be spacious enough to accommodate fractious animals without contact between them. Clients should be made to understand that, while in the reception area, their pets should be on leashes or in carrying cases.

Staff courtesy and concern for the client will be the single most important factor in making the first minutes successful. A receptionist who is smiling, helpful, knowledgeable, neatly attired, and concerned will be the key. Smoking by staff members in the reception area should not be tolerated, and a hospital policy prohibiting smoking by clients in the reception area is perfectly acceptable and may even be required by a local governmental ordinance.

Communicating Hospital Policies and Procedures

Successfully communicating hospital policies and procedures to clients will eliminate misunderstandings before they occur, will relieve you and the staff of answering countless questions many times over, and will serve to publicize many hospital services that in turn may increase business. Policies and procedures also will assist you, the manager, to better organize and manage this function of the hospital. The following ideas include effective ways to communicate hospital policies and procedures.

Hospital Information Brochure

Every new client should receive a booklet, created by the hospital, that has at least the following information:

- hospital name, address, phone numbers which are listed repeatedly and in a conspicuous manner
- doctors name(s) and specialty, if any
- extent or limitations of professional services rendered
- any nonprofessional services rendered such as boarding and grooming
- appointment hours and procedures
- emergency hours and procedures for reaching emergency coverage
- hospital policies such as receiving progress reports, visiting hospitalized animals, and discharge of patients or boarders
- payment policies—check, credit cards, deposits required on hospitalized patients
- credit privilege policies (if any)—what is required, billing charges, interest on overdue accounts, what is an overdue account

These brochures should be individually prepared for each hospital. It is probably best not to print over six months' supply so that changes can be made. Be sure not to include items such as fees that may be changed more frequently. The brochure should, in addition to being given to new clients, be readily available in the reception area for established clients and visitors. Although the hospital information brochure can represent a sizable investment, it is the best single means to establish proper communications with the clients of the hospital and will save its cost many times over in eliminating time-consuming telephone calls and conversations pertaining to the information in the brochure. It also is a very effective marketing device for the hospital.

Wall Displays

Displays in the reception area may include a roster of all doctors and staff members with titles, degrees, and specialty status; credit information pertaining to acceptance of checks, credit cards, or requirement of deposits; granting of senior citizens' discounts; and hours and emergency procedures (this should be on the wall outside the front door).

Estimate Forms

An estimate of the charges for any patient being kept in the hospital should be presented to the owner before the service is begun. Presenting the completed form to the owner will provide an opportunity to explain the service and costs to the owner and allow the owner to question the procedures before being done. This process also allows for the hospital to request a reasonable deposit if that is a hospital policy. Estimate forms can be a copy of the hospital itemized invoice, or if computerized, a computer-generated estimate. The discussion of the estimate with the owner is best done by the doctor who is in charge of the case. It should be made clear to the owner that circumstances may occur that make the estimate change, but in that case, the owner will be notified as soon as possible. The estimate should be completed in duplicate and signed by the owner with one copy going to the owner and one copy staying in the hospital with the patient's records. This copy should be kept after the animal is discharged, especially if the owner was granted credit or if there was any dispute over the charges at discharge.

Special Condition Pamphlets, Brochures and Reports

There are many sources for handouts that will give clients an opportunity to learn more about their animals' condition or health care in general. The hospital may decide to prepare its own handout on special conditions and personalize them. Handouts are available from many commercial suppliers of drugs and foods. Most of them will have some commercial message included. Handouts also may be purchased from veterinary organizations and other publishers. A major benefit of computerization is the ability to store hundreds of prewritten messages which can be generated for distribution to the client by a push of a button. All of these handouts are valuable communication instruments if time is spent by either a doctor or another staff member to explain the message and significance.

Immunization Schedules

Each new patient on its first visit for immunization should be given a schedule for future visits. Forms and brochures for this purpose are available for purchase or can be obtained free from commercial firms. This is especially important for new puppies and kittens.

Client Satisfaction Surveys

These surveys (sample in Appendix C) should be considered communication devices because they imply that the hospital cares for the client's opinion by offering a means for the client to express that opinion. Client satisfaction surveys can be done randomly throughout the year or during certain time periods. They may be mailed to clients or handed out in the office. Computerized hospitals will have an advantage in being able to easily generate a random mailing list at any time. In any case, the survey should be as private as possible if you expect honest responses from the clients.

Newsletters, computer-generated letters, and reminders will be discussed in more detail under the subject of marketing. They should all be considered as important devices for communicating hospital policies and procedures as well.

As has been emphasized throughout this manual, do not leave anything up to the memory of anyone, including yours, the staff's or the client's. Only written communications will serve this purpose.

Handling Grieving or Annoyed Clients

Inevitably there will be difficult situations to be faced by the reception staff in any animal hospital. How and when these situations are handled and resolved will test the management skills of even the most experienced and qualified managers.

The Client in Grief

This client may have concern over a sick pet, may have lost a beloved pet, or may have to make a decision about a very sick patient. The human-companion animal bond and its implications will be discussed in a future chapter. Suffice it to say that the reception staff must be sensitive to the special needs of this client. The situation should never be treated lightly as "it's only an animal," and the client should never be criticized for a show of emotion. Wherever possible, this client should be put into a quiet, nonpublic room for privacy.

Annoyed or Difficult Clients

Most of these clients will have reached this point because of a lack of communication which has created a misunderstanding that generally concerns financial matters. Proper communication will eliminate most of these situations; but when dealing with a difficult, complaining client, it will be important to listen and try to understand the source of the complaint. To immediately argue the hospital's side will only aggravate the situation. When possible, the receptionist should turn this client over to the manager who will gather the information from the client in as quiet and friendly a manner as possible. If the manager is not available or cannot resolve the problem, the matter should be immediately referred to the doctor. A very arrogant and demanding person will often become much more reasonable when the doctor is involved. A successful manager will understand this and not try to handle everything alone. The most important thing is that these situations are never resolved by confrontation and shouting matches. Letting an unreasonable client "win one" may well be worth far more than the aggravation involved.[5]

Handling Abusing or Criminal Activity

It would be nice to be able to write a manual for a perfect world in which there would never be any threat to the well-being of the staff you are managing. However, that is not the case, and as the hospital has money and drugs, it may be a target for criminal activity. There should be a hospital policy for such an occurrence. This policy should stress, above all, that the reception staff should not attempt to control the situation by themselves and should not endanger themselves in any way. If the hospital's location is such that this is a possible occurrence, consideration should be given to installation of automatic devices to contact local police. Protecting staff against violence should be a primary goal of the hospital management.

References

1. Dennis M. McCurnin, DVM, *Veterinary Practice Management*, J.B. Lippincott Co., p. 38
2. American Veterinary Medical Association, *Training Program for the Employees in the Veterinary Medical Practice*, Schaumburg, Ill.
3. Nancy Friedman, "The Telephone Doctor," videotape #5, *Five Forbidden Phrases*, The Telephone Doctor, St. Louis, Mo.
4. McCurnin, p. 26
5. McCurnin, p. 35

Chapter 4

HOSPITAL REVENUE AND FINANCIAL CONTROL

Every service transaction that takes place in the hospital will presumably create some form of revenue for the hospital. The hospital owners have determined what the services of the hospital are and what they expect to be reimbursed for providing the services. The function of the manager and staff regarding revenue and financial control will be to properly record the transaction; to collect the revenue in a manner which will, whenever possible, contribute to positive client relations; to create and collect accounts receivable if required; and to safeguard the revenue.

Recording the Transaction

In most cases, recording the fees to be charged will be done by the individual performing the service and may be done manually or by computer. If the process is manual, the actual fees will be listed on the medical record or on a charge slip created for that purpose. If the hospital is computerized, a special data form will be created which lists the services performed by the hospital (examples in Appendix D). When the services on this data form are entered into the computer, the pricing will be done automatically based on information that has been previously entered into the computer database. Whichever method is used, this is the information that is required for the transaction to be properly recorded. These charge slips and data forms should be sequentially numbered so as to facilitate accounting for each transaction.

The purpose of financial transaction recording should be to provide the client with an itemized breakdown of charges; to provide the client with a statement of the charges to be paid; and to provide the hospital bookkeeping department with the necessary information to record the income in the hospital's financial records, including information required by law.

How you record transactions will constitute the financial control system of the hospital. The method used will be determined primarily by how much financial information the hospital owners want to retain beyond what is required by law. Another consideration will be the cost of maintaining the data. The basis of the financial control system will be the manual charge slip or the computer data form. This form may have a very limited or a very extensive breakdown of services. An important consideration when designing these forms will be the need to provide the client with a meaningful, itemized breakdown of the charges. This is an absolute requirement that will minimize misunderstandings about fees.[1]

The simplest method of recording financial transactions is using a ***handwritten charge slip*** which will serve as both an itemized record and a statement of charges for the client. The total charges are recorded by the hospital in a day book which is simply a record of income. If desired by the hospital, the charge slip could be made out in duplicate with one copy retained by the hospital. This method has the advantages of being simple and less costly to implement but has the disadvantages of providing little, if any, usable information other than the amount and source. It also is very vulnerable to internal theft since there are few, if any, safeguards.

There are commercially available ***"one write" systems*** which allow the recorder to transfer information from the charge slip to the system which then creates a statement for the client as well as a financial record for the hospital from a single written entry.

Electronic cash registers can be programmed to keep track of the breakdown for each transaction and provide management with a great deal of information about the practice. Cash registers also can provide the required information for the client as well as a much higher degree of safety than the less automated methods.

Computers can provide itemized invoices, receipts, messages, and reminders about future appointments for the client and, at the same time, store information pertaining to income and inventory. You also can get a breakdown of services in every imaginable way. The ability of the computer to store information, sort it, and produce reports is mind-boggling. The value of this information will vary with each individual hospital owner. The new computer user should not be overwhelmed by the voluminous reports and database searches and forget about the safeguards that are built into the system.[2] It is important to understand that it is not necessary to have a great deal of knowledge about computers or computer training to be able to use today's computer programs.

Collecting the Revenue

The revenue of the hospital is defined as "the price of goods sold and services rendered during a given period of time" and "is equal to the inflow of cash and receivables from sales made during that period."[3] Revenue, therefore, can take many forms. Acceptance of any of the forms has some risks and creates a responsibility on the part of the person accepting. The following are forms of revenue and the concerns that should be considered by the staff member:

Currency

You can consult your bank for advice on how to spot a counterfeit bill as well as finding out if counterfeits are currently being passed in your area. Depending on the hospital's location, it may be wise not to keep large amounts of cash currency within view or reach of the clients or staff.

Checks

The hospital should have a policy on accepting checks for payment. This policy should be communicated to the client and include what identification is required and what the charge and procedure for a "bounced check" will be. Do not accept third party checks, checks made out for more than the amount owed, or post-dated checks. Always make sure that the check is signed before accepting. There are services that will guarantee checks for a fee if proper procedures are followed.

Credit Cards

The hospital will pay a bank or credit card company a percentage of the fee paid by the client with the credit card. In return, the hospital has instant cash. Credit cards must be checked for valid dates and, depending on the card, amounts over a certain figure must be authorized by an office that can be reached by telephone or by an automatic authorization device. Rejected cards usually indicate a poor credit risk. It is a good idea, in the case of a hospitalized animal where there is likely to be a large bill, to obtain the credit card numbers at the time of admission and do the credit card authorization check before the time of discharge. Then, in case the credit card does not clear, you will have time to contact the client and request an alternate form of payment. You also need to check that the card number is not on the credit card company's supplied list of stolen or delinquent cards and that the signature is the same as the one on the card. Also, the staff member performing the transaction should make sure to return the card after the processing is completed.

Accounts Receivable or Charges

Depending on whether the hospital is on a cash or accrual form of accounting (see Chapter 5), revenue earned but not collected at the time of discharge of the patient may or may not be immediate revenue for tax purposes. In any case, these revenues, which become accounts receivable, are revenue earned by the hospital and must be considered the same as currency, checks, and credit cards. Any hospital must have a policy as to whether or not they will agree to accept a charge or receivable as a method of payment for a bill rendered to a client. Hospitals that will not allow charges **must** communicate that policy to their clients **before** services are performed. If charges are accepted by the hospital, the policy should include that a credit information form specifying the terms of the agreement must be filled out on each charging client. There are examples of these forms in Appendix D. If there are to be charges for billing and interest charges, be sure to state them on the credit form and be sure that the charges comply with federal and state laws pertaining to "truth in lending" which the hospital accountant will be able to supply. These forms should be filled out in duplicate with one copy staying in the hospital and one going with the client. This form should request considerable information that will give the hospital ability to search out the client should the charge be defaulted. Merely being asked to fill out this form will, on occasion, cause the client to decide to pay the bill by check or credit card and not open a charge account.

You will need to determine what amounts can be charged without approval by either the doctor or manager, what percentage of the bill is expected to be paid at discharge, how much can be charged, and what the procedures are for aging and collecting overdue accounts receivable.[4]

To allow a client to charge a bill is, in fact, loaning the client that amount of money. If the hospital is willing to do that, you should be sure that every precaution is taken to ensure that the "loan" is repaid.

Collecting Current and Overdue Accounts Receivable

If the hospital does allow clients to charge their accounts and pay for them at a later date, there must be a record system set up for this purpose which

- identifies which clients owe the hospital money,
- generates a statement on at least a monthly basis,
- adds a billing charge or an interest charge to an account as determined by the hospital policy,
- records those accounts which are paid and enters that information into cash receipts for the day,
- "ages" accounts receivable by the number of days since the account was charged, and
- produces a report of amounts owed to the hospital both currently and overdue.

If the hospital has a manual system of financial control, the accounts receivable can be controlled by separating those transaction forms that are not paid at the time of discharge from those that are paid. This system will require careful monitoring by the responsible staff person and will require that the statements, the billing charges, interest, the aging and the payments are all recorded manually, usually onto a ledger card. Aging of the accounts in a manual system can be accomplished by using different colored "flags" on the ledger card. This process should, wherever possible, be separated from the handling of paid accounts. If the hospital is computerized, the account receivable will be recorded into the computer at the time of the transaction and a statement with a preassigned billing charge or interest will be generated by the computer. Aging of the accounts will be automatic and entering a payment in full on the account will remove the account from the receivables. The computer also will generate a report on the aging of all accounts receivable that can give an immediate picture of unpaid accounts of the hospital.

Whatever the financial control system is, the primary concern of management should be collection of the accounts in a timely manner. You can begin by sending home with the client a statement requesting that the unpaid balance be paid immediately. If a billing charge is added to the account, payment before a statement is sent should eliminate the billing charge. A return addressed envelope sent home with the statement may expedite payment.

A statement for the amount due then should be sent no later than 30 days after the charge was incurred. This first statement should be itemized and completely communicate all terms of the hospital's policy on the account such as billing charges and interest on overdue accounts. Statements are generally sent at month's end, but there may be an advantage to having the statement arrive at a time other than the bills of all of the client's other creditors. Statements should be sent consistently at the same time each month and be prompt. They should be neat and complete, giving the client an itemized accounting of the amount owed. Statements must be accurate with complete address information available. All statements should include a return addressed envelope as a convenience for the client. If the first statement is paid within 30 days after being sent, it is considered to have been paid currently. Although a billing charge may be added, interest is usually not charged on accounts paid currently.

Any account unpaid more than 30 days after a statement has been sent should be considered overdue. For this purpose, the aging of accounts is generally, but not necessarily, designated by 30 days, 60 days, 90 days, and over 90 days since the first statement was sent. The hospital should have a policy for the collection of these accounts that is definitive, consistent, and in keeping with good management. Some considerations for such a policy are as follows:

30-Day Accounts

This is the account receiving its second monthly bill. It should include an interest charge as well as a new billing charge if that is hospital policy. There is generally no major cause for concern about the account at this point but you should indicate to the client that the account is overdue. This can be accomplished by a handwritten note on the statement, a purchased sticker, or, if you are computerized, the computer will automatically print any message you want on all 30-day accounts. Hospital policy might indicate that a telephone call to certain accounts would be advisable at this time.

60-Day Accounts

This is the account receiving its third monthly bill, and nonpayment at this point should be considered a potential problem. It is time for a stronger message on the statement. A message from the doctor is often more successful than one from the manager or bookkeeper.

The hospital policy for collection of overdue accounts should include a telephone call to all clients whose accounts have not been paid by 60 days. Obviously, interest and billing charges continue to accrue.

90-Day Accounts

This will be the fourth monthly bill for this account and is cause for concern. The statement should indicate that if not paid within a specified number of days, the account will be turned over to a third party for collection unless the client has contacted the hospital with a legitimate excuse and a commitment to pay the account. A telephone call that projects a stronger message than the 60-day call should be made. Interest and billing charges continue to accrue.

Over 90-Day Accounts

Unless the client has made some attempt to contact the hospital by this time, it is suggested that the account be turned over to a collection agency. This action will cost the hospital from 35 to 50% of the account and may very well lose the client. However, waiting longer and trying to collect yourself will only make the account less collectible, and chances are that the client would not return even if you wanted that. The extent to which the hospital should go with regarding these accounts will obviously depend on several factors such as the size of the bill and the relationship with the client. If the decision is not to pursue a third party, remember that continuing to send bills is a costly procedure. It might be wiser to write off a small bill in hopes that one day the client would return to the hospital at which time the client should be made to pay the old account before being given service.

When you are calling clients with overdue accounts, you should be very careful as there are legal implications involved as well as the obvious fact that the client may be looking for an excuse not to pay the bill. All phoning to clients should be done by the office manager or bookkeeper. The person calling should have a strong, aggressive, and dominant presence on the telephone. The following are suggestions for the person making the calls:

- Have in front of you a copy of the transaction as well as the patient record that substantiates the charges. Make sure that your facts are correct.
- Get to the point about the bill. Don't start by asking how the animal is.
- Ask if the client has a dispute about the bill and, if so, get the facts. Tell the client that you will discuss the situation with the doctor and call back.
- Be prepared to give the client some options such as delayed payments over a period of time. If this is done, make the client aware that the interest and billing charges will continue and the consequences of defaulting on the agreement.
- Be sure to get some commitment from the client and be sure to follow-up on whether or not the client keeps the promise. This can be done in a manual system by making notes on a calendar to call the client if the payment has not been received.

- When calling, be aware of the client's rights under the laws of fair credit. The hospital accountant or attorney can provide that information. There are some legal situations that the caller needs to avoid (see Figure 4.1).
- You will be successful with telephone collections if the call is made before the bill is long overdue, if you communicate the hospital policy well, use good psychology, and are persistent.

Collection Agencies

The extent to which you use collection agencies is dependent primarily on the amount of the bill. Most collection agencies have a limit on the amount of the acceptable account. Most agencies only write "angry letters" that generally get angrier as they proceed. Most agencies collect as their fees a percentage of the account when it is paid but some will collect up-front fees on all accounts at the time that they start their process. Some people who owe money will pay as a result of these letters, but it would be a good idea to get from any agency you are considering a statement of effectiveness. If the agency is not successful in collecting the bill, the next step will be to use the courts to help in the collection process. Some states have small claims courts which do not require the involvement of an attorney in the collection process. Even if the process does not result in the collection of the overdue bill, there may be a judgment served against the client which could mean that the client would not be able to sell property before the judgment was cleared. Before entering into any legal process for the collection of overdue accounts, a prudent manager will weigh the costs and time involved against the chances of recovery of the owed money.

- **libelous statement**
  Never make a statement reflecting negatively on the client's character or reputation.
- **extortion**
  Never threaten to distribute bad credit information about the client.
- **invasion of privacy**
  Do not contact anyone other than the client or the immediate family, such as an employer, about the debt.
- **assault and battery**
  Never threaten any physical action if the bill remains unpaid.
- **harassment**
  Do not call at unreasonable times or at work. Do not make threatening statements about action that you might take that could be considered harassment.[5]

Figure 4.1 Tactics to avoid in bill collection

It is important to identify potential bad debts early so that they can be kept to a minimum and have the best chance of recovery. It is a fact that the more time that an account is kept open, the less the chances of collection. As previously stated, one of the major pitfalls in managing a small business is poor credit-granting practice. A well-managed business will have sound financial controls which will help protect the business against failure because of poor credit granting.

Safeguarding the Revenue

The revenues collected must be protected from loss, theft, and mishandling. This task will generally fall to the person handling the transaction. The manager's responsibility will be to establish procedures and monitor those procedures to assure the safekeeping of the revenues after collection.

First, decide on a secure place to keep the revenue as it is collected throughout the day. This place should be inaccessible to clients and all staff other than those responsible for the revenue. Then you can create a change fund that has a definite amount of money that is put in the cash drawer at the beginning of the day and is removed from the daily receipts at the end of the day.

Next, establish a check-out procedure whereby the collected revenues are added and compared to at least two other parameters such as the total of the amounts listed on the sales slips, the total on the daily log, the total on the cash register tape, or the total registered in the computer memory. This check-out should be done whenever there is a staff shift change and should be done jointly by the staff member leaving and the staff member arriving. This check-out does not have to be a final process but is meant to identify problems while all staff involved are still available. A final check-out will be done at the end of the day when daily totals will be recorded. All checks should be stamped with a "deposit only" stamp as they are collected or at least at the check-out.

After the final check-out, all collected revenue, less the established change fund, should be given to the manager or another responsible person for safe storage. There should be at least a daily deposit made into a bank. In some areas, it might be appropriate to make a night deposit and not leave the daily receipts in the hospital overnight.

Internal control by definition is "All measures used by a business to ensure against errors, waste, and fraud; to assure the reliability of accounting data; and to promote compliance with all company policies."[6] Internal control generally concerns itself with loss of revenue because of some action by a staff member. These actions could be accidental or deliberate and could involve actual money or supplies. A basic principle of internal control is that no one person should handle all phases of a transaction from beginning to end. For example, entering the transaction, collecting the revenue, handling the check-out, recording the daily receipts, making the bank deposit, and reconciling the bank statements should never be one person's responsibility.[7] Wherever possible, there should be a division of duties to prevent this occurrence. Some recommended internal control procedures concerning safeguarding hospital revenue include the following:

- All staff members handling money should be bonded.
- Staff members who handle money should be carefully selected.
- Staff members who handle money must take at least two-week vacations and allow another staff member to take over their duties.
- Charge slips or computer data forms should be serially numbered, and staff must know that the forms are being checked for missing numbers periodically. Voided slips should be kept.
- All expense payments should be paid by check or from a petty cash fund and not by taking money from the daily receipts.
- All discounts or write-offs must be approved by a doctor or the hospital manager with a signature.
- Place a sign at the cashier's desk that reads, "Please insist upon a receipt for all transactions."
- Place a sign on the exit door that reads, "Did you receive a receipt for your transaction? If not, please return to the cashier."

Employee Embezzlement

Some situations that should make a manager concerned about employee embezzlement might be a staff member with sudden, unexplained wealth; a staff member who constantly talks of money problems or asks for advances; a staff member who refuses to take vacations or share job responsibility; a staff member who frequently complains about entries made by others; check-outs that are always right; or constant client complaints about billing errors.

If you do suspect embezzlement, these are some things that you should do.

- Notify the hospital owners. Don't try to handle the situation alone.
- Rearrange staff members so that money-handling duties are shared.
- Periodically take an active part in the check-out procedure yourself.
- Contact the hospital accountant and attorney for advice, and ask for a review of the hospital records and internal control procedures.
- Inform the bonding agency.
- Make no accusations and do not talk about specific dollar amounts involved.[8]
- If guilt is determined, terminate the employee immediately. The hospital may or may not bring criminal charges, but do not think that you can trust this employee again, no matter what the reason for the embezzlement was.

Employee theft can be very costly. As a small business, animal hospitals can be particularly vulnerable because financial control systems often are relaxed for cost savings. A smaller number of employees also makes it more difficult to separate and segregate duties. Do not consider any employee fraud-proof. Whenever possible, always have two staff members handling the money, take an active part in all revenue handling activities, and do not take anything for granted.

References

1. Donald R. Dooley, "The Practice Manager," *Veterinary Practice Management*, J.B. Lippincott Co., p. 270
2. Owen E. McCafferty, CPA, "Computers: Luxury or Necessity?" *Veterinary Economics*, March 1989, p. 66
3. Walter B. Meigs and Robert F. Meigs, *Financial Accounting*, fourth edition, McGraw-Hill Book Co., p. 78
4. Priscilla K. Stockner MS, DVM, MBA, *A Practice Management Manual For Veterinarians*, Stockner and Associates, Chapter 10
5. Stockner, Chapter 10
6. Meigs and Meigs, p. 27
7. Ibid, p. 11
8. Stockner, Chapter 10

Chapter 5

ACCOUNTING AND BOOKKEEPING

Accounting Basics

Accounting is "the art of measuring, communicating, and interpreting financial activity." The purpose of accounting is to provide financial information about a business that is required by the business owners to plan and control the activities of the business. Financial information also is needed by outsiders such as creditors, potential investors or purchasers, banks, and state and federal governments for taxation purposes. The methods used by a business to keep records of its financial activities and to summarize these activities in periodic reports comprise the accounting system of the business.[1] The primary elements of accounting for any business are

- **assets**—the resources owned by the business and include buildings, land, supplies, cash on hand, and accounts receivable;
- **liabilities**—the debts or obligations of the business and include bills payable, mortgages payable, and taxes due; and
- **owners' equity**—the amount that the owners have invested in the business plus the amount of profits that have been retained in the business.

The basic accounting equation shows that assets equal liabilities plus owners' equity. In other words, owners' equity equals assets minus the debts or liabilities. A financial statement which shows the financial position of a business by summarizing the assets, liabilities, and owners' equity at a particular date is called a ***balance sheet***. A report used to evaluate the performance of a business by matching its revenue and related expenses for a particular period is called an ***income statement***. The balance sheet and the income statement together comprise the basic reports which summarize the financial position and operating results of the business and are the reports that the owners of the business will require to plan and control the activities of the hospital.[2] (There is a sample balance sheet and income statement in Appendix E.) There are numerous other reports that will be required, particularly for government, tax, and tax-related purposes. Most of this information will be available from the sources used to determine the income statement. An accounting system should be made up of a means to record the income of the hospital (an income journal) and a means to record the expenses of the hospital (an expense or disbursement journal). This recording is then entered and summarized in the book called a ***general ledger***.[3] The system can be developed to categorize the income and expenses into many areas, such as different hospital services, that would then make it possible to create a report that would give a cost accounting of individual services. A suggested Chart of Accounts, which is a logical breakdown of all hospital expenses and income, is available from the American Animal Hospital Association. The degree of categorization will be the decision of the owners as the information gained will be used primarily by them in the planning and control of the hospital. The value of the information gained must be equal to or greater than the cost of developing the reports. For tax purposes, categorization will primarily involve the expenses allocated to salaries of employees which requires that a separate payroll journal be maintained. All of the recording done in the income journal, the expense journal, the payroll journal, and the general ledger can be done with a computer. The computer will be able to break down and categorize the information and give reports based on the information in an infinite number of ways. As with the manual system, the owners will have to weigh the value of the reports to their planning with the time required to develop the information required by the computer.

Another important basic concept in accounting is the method in which income and expenses of the hospital are recorded. There are two methods known as the ***cash basis*** and the ***accrual basis***.

Accounting by the cash basis occurs when revenue is recorded when received and expenses are recorded when paid. Using the cash basis, accounts receivable would not be considered income until they were collected and accounts payable for purchases would not be considered expenses until they were actually paid.

With the accrual basis, revenue is recorded when earned and expenses recorded when incurred. With accrual accounting, an account receivable would be considered income and costs of an item in an inventory would not be considered an expense until it was actually used or resold. Accrual basis accounting matches income and expenses in the same period that they are earned and spent and gives a business a good picture of profitability which cash basis does not. However the cash basis does offer several advantages in the preparation of income tax returns.[4]

Most service businesses will use the cash basis of accounting. This decision at your animal hospital must be made with your accountant and will be affected by whether or not your business is incorporated and Internal Revenue Service (IRS) tax laws. These laws state that "no method of accounting is acceptable unless, in the opinion of the commissioner, it clearly reflects income." If the sale of inventory constitutes an appreciable source of income to the business, the IRS is likely to insist that the accrual accounting basis be used.[5]

The accounting system in most animal hospitals is developed around a bookkeeper or manager keeping the income and expense journals on a regular basis. An accountant is hired to come to the hospital periodically (usually monthly or quarterly), taking the income and expense information, putting it in the general ledger, and creating the financial statements and required government reports. A hospital with a trained bookkeeper may not require the services of an accountant more than annually. There are also accounting services which can do everything that is required to create and keep an accurate and functional accounting system. If you have any function in the area of accounting, you should be familiar with the basics of accounting and the terminology of accounting which has been called "the language of business." Appendix E has a glossary of commonly used accounting terms.

Duties of a Bookkeeper

The bookkeeper's duties basically involve recording the transactions into the journals and ledgers. While the bookkeeping function is relatively simple, it does take time and some skill and should not be given to just anyone with free time. The job should be handled by as few people as possible to achieve conformity and continuity in the record keeping. Bookkeepers do not require degrees or licenses but most will have taken business and accounting courses in a college or trade school. If your hospital is computerized, the bookkeeper should have a basic knowledge of computers as well. In most animal hospitals, many duties beyond the recording of transactions will fall onto the individual designated as the bookkeeper. The following is a partial list of the tasks that could be part of the job description of a bookkeeper in an animal hospital:

- Maintaining payroll records and preparing and distributing payroll. This requires a method of properly recording the hours worked by the employees, such as a time sheet or time cards, and the knowledge of the proper means to determine the appropriate withholdings from the salaries.
- Preparing, at the designated times, the required state and federal reports pertaining to payroll. These reports involve FICA, withholding taxes, insurance payments, and other money due to the taxing agencies and require submission of the money withheld from the employee salaries as well as the employer portions. In all cases, late submission of these reports will involve penalties. There will be reports requiring weekly, monthly, quarterly, and annual submission depending on the size of the payroll. The bookkeeper should be aware of what reports are required and when they are due to be filed as well as the reports and forms that are required to be on file in the hospital. If the bookkeeper is responsible for the payment of funds payable to the federal and state governments and the funds are not paid, the bookkeeper may be held liable for that money even though there is no ownership or financial interest in the business.
- Verifying daily income reports and preparing and making daily bank deposits. The bookkeeper also may be responsible for maintaining the accounts receivable of the hospital, including recording payments.
- Preparing checks for the owner's signature for the payment of accounts payable. Each statement should be signed or initialed by a responsible party showing that the materials have been received or the service has been completed and that the price has been

verified. In most animal hospitals, the statement should be approved for payment by the hospital owner before the payment is prepared.

- Maintaining the checkbook and verifying the balances on a regular basis.
- Maintaining the necessary information and recording all of the data required to keep a current income journal, disbursements journal, payroll journal, and general ledger.
- In some cases, a bookkeeper may be assigned the task of preparing the income statement, balance sheet, and annual tax returns. In most cases, however, these tasks will become the responsibility of the accountant.
- In some hospitals, the bookkeeper might be responsible for maintaining employee personnel files, recording vacation and sick days, and determining employee benefits as directed by hospital policy.

The bookkeeper's duties are very sensitive and whenever any one person records entries, pays bills, and receives incoming cash, there will be more than the usual opportunity for employee embezzlement. For this reason, the bookkeeper should be carefully chosen, bonded, and closely monitored. The principles of internal control, as discussed in Chapter 4, should be considered and closely followed.

As previously mentioned, there are bookkeeping services to do most of the duties of an in-house bookkeeper. They are usually computerized and will supply the hospital with a myriad of computerized reports. They are efficient and obviously know when reports are due and eliminate the possibility of penalty for a late report. They may offer an accountant's service as well; however, for purposes of internal control, it may be advisable to separate the bookkeeping and accounting functions. They are expensive and since they are "out-of-house," that means that many of your records are also out of the hospital. The service tends to be impersonal and serves little function as a source of information for planning purposes.

An out-of-house service that should be considered by any animal hospital with 10 or more employees is a payroll service. After giving the payroll service basic information on the employee such as name, social security number, number of dependents, hourly or weekly salary, and any voluntary withholding, the service will require that for each payroll period they be supplied with the number of hours worked in that period by each employee. They will then prepare the payroll checks, making the requested and required withholdings, and prepare the required tax reports for the hospital to submit. It is also possible to have the required employee taxes automatically impounded from the hospital checking account and sent to the responsible agencies.

The Hospital Accountant

Accounting, as opposed to bookkeeping, includes the design of accounting systems, preparation of financial statements, audits, cost studies, development of forecasts, income tax work, computer applications to accounting processes, and the analysis and interpretation of accounting information as an aid in making business decisions. Accountants are professionals with extensive education in their field and are expensive. A certified public accountant (CPA) is an accountant who has a license to practice in a given state based on taking and passing a vigorous examination and having extensive experience. A CPA is licensed to audit financial records and to certify that those records are true. A certified, audited financial statement may be required in many financial transactions such as acquiring large bank loans or the sale of a business. A CPA may also represent the hospital in an IRS audit. An accountant who is not a CPA may represent a client before the IRS if they are admitted as an enrolled agent before doing so.

Every animal hospital should have the regular services of an accountant. However, the accountant should not be hired to do bookkeeping. The optimum arrangement would be for a bookkeeper or bookkeeping service to prepare all journals up to and including the general ledger. All monthly and quarterly reports and required disbursements for a quarterly inspection would be done by the accountant. The accountant would prepare quarterly financial statements and arrange a conference to discuss them with the owner at that time. At the end of the fiscal year, the accountant will prepare the year-end financial statements and the annual tax reports. Your accountant should be able to help the hospital owners and manager with tax planning, offer advice on short-term and long-term financial strategies, provide financial reports, help to prepare loan applications, and customize the internal control procedures. An accountant's major function should be to help the hospital obtain financial success. Owners and hospital managers should use a knowledgeable accountant and ask for advice. Be prepared to share your plans and objectives with the accountant and clearly explain your expectations. If the accountant's advice is properly given and properly followed, it should create a profit which will more than offset their fees.

To find an accountant, ask your banker, lawyer, or other business colleagues for recommendations. It is important that the personality of the accountant be well-suited to the personalities and management styles of both the owner and the manager. Experience with other animal hospitals is helpful but not necessary if the accountant takes a serious and personal interest in your hospital. Large accounting firms will give you specialists in many fields, but you are not likely to get the same personal service as with a smaller firm. Before hiring an accountant, interview at least two and find out what their commitment to servicing your hospital is. Get referrals from at least two of their clients of two to five years. The American Institute of Certified Public Accountants publishes a free pamphlet, "101 Questions to Ask Your CPA." To get a copy, send a stamped, self-addressed envelope to AICPA, 1211 Avenue of the Americas, New York, NY 10036.

Accounting and Bookkeeping by Computer

The hospital accounting system and the journals and ledgers that make it up can all be part of a computer software program. The accounting system may be separate by itself or it may be integrated with daily receipting, with accounts receivable, and with inventory purchases and sales. The integrated system is preferable because a great deal of the data required by the accounting system is entered as a single entry for another purpose. The computer accounting system will be capable of revenue and disbursement breakdown by as many categories as the hospital owners wish. These breakdowns can be by services and by the doctor who rendered the service. As a general rule, the accounting system will have a chart of accounts which will identify the income and expenses for the computer in a constant and uniform manner. The computer will generate the journals; create the general ledger; generate transaction analysis based on the breakdowns; give daily, monthly, and yearly analysis of income and expenses to compare with past periods; create required payroll reports; and even prepare checks for accounts payable and payroll. The computer could also be programmed to create the hospital's financial statements on as frequent a basis as needed. A computer accounting system will rarely eliminate the need for a hospital bookkeeper and may even require a bookkeeper with knowledge of computerized bookkeeping. If properly used, the computer should require less time for the bookkeeper while making that time more productive. A computer will never eliminate the need for an accountant but will give the accountant and the hospital owner much more information more frequently and faster for management decisions and planning. Although there are other advantages to computerizing an animal hospital that may generate a more identifiable return on the investment in a computer such as target marketing, reminder processing, inventory control, and accounts receivable tracking, the use of a computer for accounting and bookkeeping will serve a very useful purpose in an animal hospital.

References

1. Walter B. Meigs and Robert F. Meigs, *Financial Accounting*, fourth edition, McGraw-Hill Book Co., p.1
2. Dennis H. Tootelian and Ralph M. Gaedeke, *Small Business Management*, Scott Foresman and Co., p. 468
3. Meigs and Meigs, p. 104
4. Reg. 1.446-1 (a) (1) Internal Revenue Service Code, 1986
5. Meigs and Meigs, p. 6

Chapter 6

MEDICAL RECORDS

What Are Medical Records?

Medical records are an important tool in the practice of veterinary medicine. They serve as a basis for planning patient care and as a means of communication between members of the hospital staff. They furnish documentary evidence of the patient's illness, care, and treatment. They serve as a basis of review, study, and evaluation of the medical care rendered by the hospital.[1] Although the patient's medical history and treatment chart are usually the primary components of a medical record, the following medical and business documents are also considered medical records:

- client registration forms
- appointment books
- client consent forms
- radiographs
- estimate sheets
- financial records
- anesthesia records
- telephone consultations
- controlled drug logs
- surgery logs
- radiology logs
- laboratory logs

- patient discharge records
- electrocardiograms and other electrical examinations
- laboratory reports
- necropsy reports[2]

Every animal hospital has to establish what type of medical record system it will have. Choices will range between recording information directly onto a medical record card in a continuous manner; recording information on separate sheets and keeping all of the sheets in a folder; or keeping all of the information in a computer.

There are several card and folder systems specifically designed for use in animal hospitals which are available commercially. Regardless of the type of system used, the following criteria should apply to all records of the examination and treatment rendered to animals in an animal hospital:

- There should be a separate record on each animal.
- The record should be written in a scientific manner.
- The record must be kept as a legal document that will be admissible in a court of law.
- The record should provide for easily retrievable information on the patient.
- The record **must** be accurate and legible. The value of medical records is in direct proportion to the thoroughness and accuracy with which they are compiled.[3]

What Should Be Included on a Medical Record?

Each medical record should include the following information either recorded as a permanent part of the record at the time of the first visit by the patient or recorded at the time of each visit or hospitalization.

- **Client identification**—Record the name, home address, home telephone number, work address, and work telephone number of the client.
- **Patient identification**—Identify each patient by species, breed, sex, name, color, markings, and age or date of birth. The patient's weight should be recorded at each visit.
- **Previous medical history**—This should include any problems reported and treatment given to the patient before the initial visit.
- **Vaccination history**—This should be updated each time that the patient receives a vaccination.

- **The primary complaint**—This should be an accurate history gathered from the client of the reasons that the patient was brought to the hospital.
- **Physical examination**—A brief report of the results of the examination completed at each visit with a listing of the problems encountered.
- **Diagnosis or a list of possible diagnoses**—When a definitive diagnosis is made, it should be recorded as such.
- **Treatment given or prescribed**—All drugs used and doses should be carefully included.
- **Laboratory reports**—All laboratory tests performed and all abnormal findings should be included as a permanent part of the medical record.
- **Radiographic and electrocardiogram reports**
- **Consultation reports**
- **Prognosis**—Whenever possible, the doctor's evaluation of the eventual outcome should be recorded.
- **Surgical record**—This should be a comprehensive record of all surgical procedures (including the type and dosage of anesthetics used) and identification of the surgeon.
- **Dental records**—Record carefully any extractions as well as corrective procedures taken.
- **Necropsy reports**—This should include laboratory tissue reports.

Methods of Organizing Medical Records

Information on a medical record can be organized in three ways. The first is a ***source-oriented medical record*** which consists of data entered on the record from various sources in chronological order for each office visit or period of hospitalization. The method of recording the data can be individualized to suit the wants and needs of the veterinarian. Most entries are written as they come to the mind of the writer. Source-oriented medical records can be effective if they are organized and legible and the information is easily retrievable. They also should include a list of the problems the patient has been treated for.

The second method is a ***problem-oriented medical record*** (POMR) that is chronologically ordered according to each problem that has been identified. The record has four sections, beginning with the defined database which includes the chief complaint, the patient profile, history, physical examination, and laboratory and radiology reports. Next is the problem list with its three sections—the major problem list, a minor problem list, and a medication table. The third section is the plans section which includes written discussion of further diagnostic procedures, therapy, and client education. Finally, there is the progress section written in the "SOAP" format. SOAP is an acronym which stands for

> **S**—subjective information, including the presenting complaint and the history
> **O**—objective information, including the exam and laboratory findings
> **A**—assessment of the data, including a provisional diagnosis
> **P**—plan being made for further diagnostic studies and for treatment and possible surgery

Although POMR makes data very easy to retrieve and permits a rapid evaluation of the condition of the patient at any given time, it is very time consuming to compose and for this reason will probably not be the method of choice in many animal hospitals.[4,5]

The third choice is a ***combination of source- and problem-oriented methods*** which is the most appropriate way to organize the information on the medical record. Using this method, the medical record would employ a major problem list and a vaccination history; organize the initial examination into the SOAP format; and follow the case on a daily basis with a source format.

Filing Medical Records

Noncomputerized medical records are kept on cards or in folders and can be filed either alphabetically or numerically. The alphabetical method has the advantage of not requiring a cross-reference file and its easier to organize. Its disadvantages are that the person doing the work must know how to spell or there may be the possibility of lost or misfiled records. The alphabetical system also can be confusing with clients with the same names.

With the numerical system, each client is assigned a number. That number can come from a consecutive list or use the client's telephone or Social Security number. The number must be referenced to the client's name in a cross-reference file. The numerical system's advantages are that it is easier to read, spelling is not a factor, and it can be combined with color tabs to give a quick visual method of filing and retrieval. The disadvantages are the need for a cross-reference file; it can be more time-consuming to find a file; and telephone numbers, if used, can change.

Retrieval of medical records can be enhanced with either system with the use of signaling devices. Signaling devices can be colored metal or plastic tabs attached to the record or colored stickers attached to folders. They are used to make retrieval of certain files easier. Signals on medical records can be used to designate certain animals that require vaccinations, dentistry, or other regular preventive services at specified time intervals in order to send out reminders. Use signals also to flag clients who owe money—certain colored tabs or stickers could be used to denote the number of days that the account is overdue. Signals also can indicate clients to whom estimates have previously been given and the last time that the animal was in the hospital in order to purge the files periodically or to contact those clients who had not visited the hospital in a specific period of time.

Logs Commonly Used in Animal Hospitals

Logs are a continuous record, generally kept chronologically, for one particular service. They are kept for legal reasons, in the case of the use of narcotics, or for information retrieval reasons and technique comparison, as in the case of a surgery or radiology log. They also may be kept as a part of the patient medical record with a reference in the record to the log, or they may be kept for economic and financial data to justify certain procedures and the amount of work done in certain areas. Some of the more common logs kept are listed below in Figure 6.1 and there are samples of most of these logs in Appendix F.

- **Surgery Log** This log should have a record of the patient, the type of surgery, the weight of the animal, the name of the surgeon, and any unusual occurrence.
- **Anesthetic Log** This may be a separate log or combined with the surgery log. It should be a record of the type and amount of all anesthetic materials used. Anesthetic deaths or serious complications also should be recorded.
- **Controlled Drug Log** A sample of this log is not included in Appendix F since laws pertaining to the recording of any narcotics used in the hospital are very specific and may vary. Please check with your federal, state, or provincial governments for the specific laws in your area.
- **Radiology Log** This log should have patient information, the area of the body radiographed, the instrument settings, and the radiographic findings.
- **Laboratory Log** This log can be as extensive, as far as what tests are included, as the hospital wishes. The purpose of this log is primarily to demonstrate the amount of work done (i.e., the number of heartworm tests, fecals, or the amount of laboratory work done in-house versus out-of-house).
- **Euthanasia Log** If narcotics are used for euthanasia, this log, in addition to giving retrieval information, would be a legal requirement.
- **Syringe and Medical Waste Log** This is a requirement in some states and may soon be required in all.

Figure 6.1 Types of logs

Legal Implications of Medical Records

There will be questions pertaining to ownership, possession, access, confidentiality, and retention of medical records. There also will be questions pertaining to ownership and retention of radiographs. There will be questions and problems relating to lost medical records. All of these questions may have different answers depending on the state or province. The hospital attorney should be consulted in most of these cases. Also, an excellent resource for these questions is Chapter 14 of *Law and Ethics of the Veterinary Profession* by James F. Wilson, DVM, JD.[6]

Computerized Medical Records

Most computerized animal hospitals will have the capability of maintaining medical records as well as financial records in the computer. The decision to use or not use that capability is one that must be made by each hospital and its owners and managers. Some hospitals will keep only patient information, vaccination history, and a list of the patients' major problems on the computer, with the remainder of the medical record kept on a record card or in a folder system. Another hospital may decide to keep all logs on the computer. Still another hospital may have its entire medical record on the computer with no written records whatsoever in the hospital. Although all integrated software packages will have the capacity for medical records, they will all differ in the mechanics of keeping the records. The pros and cons of computerized medical records are discussed in Figures 6.2 and 6.3.

- Takes up less space—no large filing cabinets required.
- Information on the records is more consistent, especially when more than one doctor is involved, allowing for quicker and more exact data retrieval.
- Takes less time to input the information into the computer than to write it onto a record.
- Records always will be legible.
- Ease of accessing information about the medical history of the patient will make target marketing for such services as geriatric workups, dental services, any repeat visits, and vaccination reminders much easier than with a manually written system.
- Accessing medical records and other information in different locations. This is particularly necessary if the hospital has more than one outpatient location.

Figure 6.2 Advantages of computerized medical records

- When the computer is out of service, i.e., in an electrical outage, there will be no records.
- Records can be "lost" in the computer if the system fails.
- Computerized records can be altered and may not be admissible as court evidence. This question has been considered in many states and provinces. It appears that if the court is satisfied that the information on the computer record is trustworthy, if the entries have been made at or near the time the event occurred, and if the computer is recognized as standard equipment in the business, then the computerized records will be admissible as evidence.
- Computer records won't accommodate detailed descriptions. Codes and set phrases will be used.
- Medical records on the computer require that the computer have a much greater storage capacity than would otherwise be required.

Figure 6.3 Disadvantages of computerized medical records

References

1. American Animal Hospital Association, *Standards for AAHA Hospitals*, Denver, Colo., p. 5
2. James F. Wilson, DVM, JD, *Law and Ethics of the Veterinary Profession*, Priority Press Ltd., p. 317
3. American Animal Hospital Association, *Medical Records Manual, Denver, Colo., p. 2.02*
4. Wilson, p. 318
5. *Medical Records Manual*, p. 2.02
6. Wilson, p. 325

Chapter 7

INVENTORY CONTROL AND MANAGEMENT

Inventory is defined as all goods owned and held for sale or use in the regular course of business.[1] Inventory control is defined as the process whereby the need to maintain sufficient inventory to meet the hospital's needs is weighed against the cost of carrying inventory to arrive at an appropriate inventory level.[2] As a hospital manager, there is no other area in the hospital where you can contribute more to increasing the hospital's profit than in inventory control and management. The goals of inventory control and management include the following:

- patients and clients have the necessary medications and supplies when they need them;
- drugs and supplies turn over four to eight times per year (turnover will be explained later);
- staff can easily order, stock, and dispense the needed items;
- controlled drugs are properly monitored and handled; and
- a reasonable profit is realized.[3]

To accomplish these goals, it will be necessary to have a workable inventory system in the hospital.

Inventory System: What Should It Include?

An inventory system in the hospital may be manual or computerized. In either case, it is absolutely necessary to have one inventory manager and to use inventory control cards.

The individual who is assigned as an inventory manager will order and stock supplies and maintain inventory records. This individual should be the only person in the hospital who has contact with the sales people and probably should not be a veterinarian. The right individual in this position is the key to an effective inventory system. There will be less, if any, duplication of items and less drugs purchased that are not efficacious. Excessive stock will be avoided; problem orders will be monitored; and problem vendors will be easily identified.[4] With new drugs, a good procedure to follow is that no new drug should be ordered until it is discussed by the doctors in a staff meeting.

The inventory control card system can be a manual one (sample in Appendix G) or a computer software program. The inventory manager must record for each item purchased the following information:

- **item**—size, color, strength, dispensing format, trade name or generic name, hospital code name or number, if used
- **suppliers**—name, address, telephone number, hospital account number, catalog number
- **quantity**—number and date ordered and number and date received
- **reordering**—maximum reorder number and minimum reorder point which is when quantity on hand reaches a specified amount
- **costs**—item, tax, shipping
- **location in hospital**—is the item used in the hospital or dispensed; number on hand at certain intervals
- **price to client**—formula for determining price

If the hospital's accounting system is set up to allocate certain supply expenses to certain hospital services or areas (profit centers), this control card or program also should have the ability to make that allocation.

What Should the Inventory System Do?

The inventory manager and an effective inventory system should accomplish a variety of important functions. The inventory system will ensure that all items used in the hospital are available at all times and will signal the manager when an item should be reordered. The system will enable a hospital to stock adequate supplies without investing unnecessary capital as well as enable a hospital to allocate expenses of supplies to different profit centers. The manager will be able to assess an accurate value of the inventory at any given time and especially at year end as required by tax laws. The system can provide information on where the item is available at the least cost and how to order it, reduce costs or ordering, and identify back orders and when they are expected. It also will enable the hospital to do cost-effective purchasing by identifying such things as seasonal usage that allows for purchasing at optimal times and at optimal quantities. An effective system allows for outdated items to be identified and removed from the inventory, ensures that items contracted at specific prices are delivered and billed at those prices, passes on any increased purchase costs to the client immediately, and helps control pilferage. Above all, an effective inventory system must be simple to use.

How to Maintain the Inventory System

Whether the inventory system is manual or computerized, the inventory manager will be required to closely monitor the supplies as to the amount on hand, the usage, and whether they are outdated or not. The inventory manager, using a manual system, should have a job description which includes the following responsibilities:

- To create and maintain an inventory control card on every item purchased and used in the hospital. This may be restricted to items used for the care and treatment of patients or may include stationery, office forms, supplies, sundries, equipment, and furnishings.
- To constantly review inventory cards as well as drug supplies on shelves and other areas in the hospital to determine if an item has reached its reorder point. There may also be a "want list" created to allow others to record items that are in low supply.
- To be familiar with and monitor usage of drugs and supplies, especially seasonal items, so as to order these supplies at the proper time in sufficient quantities.
- To know the schedules of sales people who visit the hospital in order to be able to order all items at one time from a minimum number of sources.
- To record on the inventory card the information pertaining to the order for that item.
- To note on the inventory card when the order is received and the receipt, including any price changes. Items ordered but not received (back orders) should be treated as not received. The packing slip or invoice should be noted as being in order or not and given to the person responsible for payment.
- To stock the items on the shelves so that the newly received items are used after current stock. This is especially important with items that are dated.
- To monitor dated materials periodically and remove outdated items from the shelves. This can be done by checking each item or may be done by coding the items with colored stickers that denote a month in which the item will be outdated. Some suppliers will allow outdated materials to be returned for credit.

- To do a physical inventory of the items most used in the hospital at least every three months, and do a complete inventory of all supplies at least yearly.

In a large hospital using a manual system, two additional items should probably be added to this job description

- To maintain a purchase order system that traces every order placed from determination of need to payment. One copy would go to the company with which the order is placed, another copy kept and then checked against the company's packing slip when the order is received. This copy then is sent to the bookkeeper to check against the invoice before payment. Most business supply stores will have purchase order forms available.
- To maintain a supply inventory and working inventory. Drugs and supplies would be signed out of the supply inventory to specific work areas in the hospital that would be responsible for the working inventory. For example, if the treatment area was to be allocated 25 doses of vaccine or a bottle of prednisolone, these items, for supply inventory purposes, would be considered used and subject to reorder. Care must be taken not to have excessive amounts of drugs and supplies in areas other than the main supply inventory.

Using a Computer

If the hospital uses a computerized inventory system, everything stated above would still be done except that many jobs would be done by or simplified by the computer. For example, in a computer system where items are removed from the inventory as they are shown as being sold or used on the customer receipting process, the computer will be able to record the number and the value of the inventory by item or as a total.

If programmed with a reorder point for each inventory item, the computer will keep track of usage and signal the inventory manager when an item has reached the reorder point.

When the inventory manager enters the receipt of an order and the price of a given item has changed, the computer will automatically compute a new resale price for that item, based on a previously programmed formula.

The computer is capable of creating a purchase order for a supplier based on its knowledge of what items have reached reorder points and from which suppliers these items are purchased.

There are services available that can be accessed by computer that will ensure that any ordered item is ordered from the supplier with the lowest price. The computer also could place the order.

The inventory system can provide hospital personnel with information needed to prevent errors in medication such as dosages, contraindications, etc.

Hidden Costs of Inventory

A simple solution to prevent the hospital inventory from ever running out of any item would be to purchase and maintain an inventory of all items that are excessive in comparison to use. There is, however, a problem associated with this "simple" solution and that is the cost of inventory. In addition to the actual cost to purchase the inventory item, there are other costs which make up the hidden costs of inventory management. Some of these are costs of ordering, handling, and storage of the item; protection of the item against heat and cold; and insurance and taxes. Other hidden costs are obsolescence and spoilage if not used or sold immediately and loss of earning opportunities for the money that has been used to pay for the inventory.

All of these costs increase the longer any inventory item is held in the hospital. It should be obvious that optimal inventory control will involve an astute policy of purchasing inventory so as to minimize these hidden costs while at the same time having the items required to operate the hospital available at all times.

How, When, and How Much to Order

When contemplating any type of inventory control program, it is very important to consider an item called Pareto's Law or the "80-20 rule." The 80-20 rule says that 20 percent of the inventory accounts for 80 percent of the sale or use. This rule tells the inventory manager to determine what items make up this 20 percent and be sure that these items are given special consideration. The other 80 percent should not be forgotten but care should be taken not to overstock them.

The key to an efficient and effective ordering policy rests with the inventory manager's familiarity with the suppliers of the needed items and a knowledge of the usage of the items to be ordered which should be available if the inventory card is properly utilized. Here are some suggestions of how and when to order inventory for an animal hospital.

- Know when suppliers' representatives will be visiting the hospital. Being ready will save time.
- Keep a list of the items that are due to be reordered from each supplier. Prepare purchase orders if they are to be used. Try to order an entire month's requirement from each supplier.
- Deal with as few suppliers as possible. This will save time in ordering, unpacking, handling, invoice checking, and bill paying. This also can make the hospital a more important customer to those suppliers and give them more incentive to provide excellent service.
- Anticipate seasonal ordering such as flea treatments in the spring.

- Try to order as much as possible during the last five days of the month. Most companies "close their books" about the 25th of the month so items purchased after that day will not be billed until the first of the following month.
- Only call in orders in emergencies. Mistakes are too easily made. Use a facsimile machine if it is available.
- Try not to order small quantities that may bear additional shipping charges.

Determining Quantities

How much to order of each item is obviously the most important question to be answered in inventory control. Too little of an item creates shortages and causes lost sales and services while too much of an item increases the expense of inventory and costs additional dollars to the hospital. The key to knowing how much to order is to establish for each item a reorder point and a maximum inventory number.

The reorder number for each item will be determined by the number used, how fast it is used, and how long it takes to order and receive the item. This number should assure the hospital that if that number is available at the time of order, that there will be at least one left when the new order is received.

You can establish an inventory turnover for the entire hospital inventory. This turnover number is determined by dividing the total dollar amount spent on purchases of drugs and supplies in a year by the average dollar value of the inventory maintained in the hospital at any given time. This number tells you how many times in a given year your inventory "turns over" or is totally used. For example, if the total spent for drugs and supplies in a year was $120,000 and the value of the inventory was $20,000, the turnover number would be six or every two months. The higher this number is, the more efficient is the inventory control. There is no accurate standard but a turnover of eight to 10 (35 to 45 days) would probably be a target range for most hospitals.[5] Too high a turnover number, although financially efficient via a faster return on inventory investment, also has the danger of creating shortages. After establishing the hospital inventory turnover number, establish the same turnover number with as many of the inventory items (especially the 20 percent) as possible. This number will allow the inventory manager to determine the maximum inventory number for each item. Remember this number will not be constant over a year's time for seasonal items.

There is a formula that may be used to determine what the "economic ordering quantity" or the optimum quantity of any one item to be ordered each time an order is placed. This formula is EOQ = 2FS/CP when

EOQ = economic ordering quantity

F = fixed costs of placing and receiving an order

S = annual sales in units

C = carrying costs (hidden costs) expressed as a percentage of inventory value

P = purchase price per unit of inventory[6]

It would not make sense to apply this formula to every item carried in a hospital inventory. However, it could be used to purchase very high use items.

If the inventory manager develops an efficient inventory system, understands inventory control and the costs of creating and maintaining an inventory, and uses meaningful data established from past usage of each item, it is possible to estimate very accurately what the maximum inventory number should be. The important test of this system will be an inventory turnover of six or higher and an absolute minimal number of shortages of any item.

Other Means of Inventory Control

There are many other means that you may try to effect additional savings and profits from inventory. First of all beware of deals that offer discounts for purchasing large quantities of an item. The discount must be sufficient to offset the costs of maintaining the inventory until it is sold. Few deals ever justify purchasing more than a three-month supply of any item.

By purchasing an item at the very end or beginning of the month, the hospital will not receive a bill for that item for at least 30 days after receipt. You then will have the ability to sell or use the item for those 30 days. If your turnover number is six (your average inventory is used up in 60 days) and you have had 30 days to sell the item before you need to pay for it and if you have doubled the purchase price as your selling price, what has occurred? You have already received from the sale of a 30-day supply of the item (one half of the order) the amount of money that you now must pay the company for the 60-day supply. This means that you have not used any of the hospital's money to have that item available in the hospital. This example, although simple, should not be difficult to duplicate with most of the 20 percent of the 80-20 items in the hospital inventory.

You may want to have the drug and supply distributor maintain the inventory for you. Many distributors will be willing to agree that if the hospital purchases a certain amount of an item over a specified period of time, the distributor will keep the product in the warehouse and ship and bill your hospital either on a preset schedule or as your hospital requests. This agreement generally offers a generous discount and eliminates most of the hidden costs of inventory.

Comparison shop for supplies, especially sundries like toilet paper and towels or printed forms and stationery. Most of these items can be purchased for much less at certain times of the year when the vendor is not as busy. This may be the one exception to the three-month rule. If your hospital uses large quantities of specially printed forms, it could be advantageous to have several firms bid on preparing them.

For equipment purchases, there is a definite economic advantage to having bids from several vendors. A necessary prerequisite is to know exactly what you want and the specifications for the equipment.

Inventory from an Accounting Standpoint

Under the accrual basis of accounting, inventory becomes an asset of the business as soon as it is received. Under the cash basis, inventory becomes an asset as soon as the bill is paid. In either case, inventory is always a very large item on the asset side of the balance sheet. Although inventory is an asset, it is nonproductive unless sold or used and consequently it costs money until sold or used. In a veterinary practice, excessive inventory ties up funds, requires storage, and represents loss if it becomes outdated or unsalable. An effective and efficient inventory control program will produce profit for any business.

References

1. Walter B. Meigs and Robert F. Meigs, *Financial Accounting*, fourth edition, McGraw-Hill Book Co., p. 336
2. Dennis H. Tootelian and Ralph M. Gaedke, *Small Business Management*, Scott Foresman and Co., p. 741
3. Priscilla K. Stockner, MS, DVM, MBA, "Inventory Control Equals Hidden Profits," *Trends Magazine*, Vol. III, No. 2, American Animal Hospital Association, p. 24
4. Stuart D. Forney, "Inventory, Prescriptions and Drugs," *Veterinary Practice Management*, J.B. Lippincott Co., p. 347
5. Robert E. Froehlich, DVM, MBA, *Successful Financial Management for the Veterinary Practice*, American Animal Hospital Association, Denver, Co., p. 23
6. Marc Schapiro, MS, MBA, "Inventory Management and Control," a lecture given at the 54th Annual Meeting of the American Animal Hospital Association, Phoenix, Ariz., March 1987

Chapter 8

THE HUMAN-COMPANION ANIMAL BOND

Much has been written and said about the subject of the human-companion animal bond. A list of pertinent resources on the subject is in Appendix H. These books and other materials should be available in all animal hospitals for use by staff and clients. Any staff person who has responsibility for the care of the animal patients and the relationship of that patient to its owner should be familiar with the resources noted.

A good hospital manager should be aware of the relationship of the human-companion animal bond and a successful, well-managed animal hospital. Dr. William F. McCulloch, a pioneer in the study of the relationship between people and their pets, said, "In addition to caring for animal patients, today's veterinarian is responsible, directly or indirectly, for maintaining and improving the physical, mental, and emotional well being of his or her clients.... Society has only recently begun to realize that veterinarians in companion animal practice are more than luxury practitioners serving those who can afford pets. They are increasingly applying their veterinary skills, knowledge, and resources to the protection and improvement of human health."[1]

The Human-Companion Animal Bond and Normal Hospital Activity

The human-companion animal bond is defined as a continuous, bidirectional relationship between a human and an animal that brings a significant benefit to a central aspect of the lives of each, which is in some sense voluntary, and in which each party treats the other not just as something entitled to respect and benefit in its own right but also as an object of admiration, trust, devotion, or love.[2] Within the normal activities regularly encountered in an animal hospital, there are activities which require an understanding of this special relationship.

- advice on a new pet purchase
- leaving a pet in the hospital for treatment or surgery
- any treatment or handling procedure where the pet might experience pain or fright
- treatment and handling of pets specially trained to provide assistance for the blind, hearing impaired, or emotionally disturbed
- involvement with programs designed for pet visitation to nursing and group homes or other pet assistance programs
- animal behavior problems both in the hospital and as a concern for the owner's ability and willingness to keep the animal
- advice to pet owners with family members allergic to animals
- treatment of conditions and diseases that are contagious to owners
- advice to pet owners who must relocate to places where they may not take their pets
- request to provide gratuitous or low-cost veterinary services to the needy
- discussion of pet care and needs with and/or in the presence of young children in the family
- recommending euthanasia to an owner with a seriously ill or injured pet
- agreeing or not agreeing to perform euthanasia on an animal for financial, behavioral, or other reasons when the animal's life was not in danger
- accidental death of a pet

In all of these cases, the veterinarians and the staff members can satisfy the needs of the owners and build a strong relationship, destroy that relationship, or not allow it to develop by being insensitive to the feelings of the client that are built upon the bond between the client and the animal. To a great extent, how veterinarians and staff assist pet owners in each of these situations will relate to their own beliefs and values. There also will often be ethical considerations and values involved, and no client should expect these to be compromised. However, any individual working in any capacity in an animal hospital must have an understanding of the human-companion animal bond. Those who are insensitive or skeptical of the bond should not be employed in any capacity.

The Staff's Role When an Animal Dies or Euthanasia is Necessary

Although all of the conditions that involve an understanding of the human-companion animal bond in the daily operation of an animal hospital are important, the one condition that will cause the most concern and involvement with the staff is the death of a pet. Euthanasia of a seriously injured or terminally ill pet will be the decision of the owner after consultation with the veterinarian. Although nonveterinary staff members should never take a role in this process, they are often asked by the owner what their feelings are. Grieving owners often relate more directly to staff members than to the veterinarians at this point. It may be that the veterinarian has become the "bad guy" because of an inability to cure the animal and now the veterinarian wants to "kill" it. The staff role at this point has to be to reinforce the decision and assure the owner that everything possible has been done for the pet. If a staff member has any personal doubt about the veterinarian's recommendation, that person should leave the room. Figure 8.1 has a list of procedures for veterinarians and staff to follow prior to and following euthanasia of a pet. If the animal has died in the hospital or in an accident, those steps relating to grief, visitation with the body, disposal of the body, and letters and records should be followed.

There are several reasons why veterinarians and staff should be sensitive to an owner's needs during the crisis of having a beloved pet euthanized. Helping the client resolve the grief of losing a pet is one further act of kindness that the staff can perform for a client. The staff also may be the only people with sufficient understanding of what is going on inside the client's mind to be of any help. Frequently, even other family members may not be experiencing the same emotions and are unable to understand what is happening. According to a study for the Pet Food Institute, 15 percent of former pet owners do not replace lost pets because going through the grief process was too painful. Finally, letting a client leave the hospital with unresolved anger will be hazardous to the reputation of the hospital.[3]

Although the veterinarian and staff will be primarily concerned with the emotions of the clients during the loss of a pet, there is always a very real possibility that staff members and veterinarians will be emotionally affected as well. Veterinarians and staff should be encouraged to speak openly with each other about their feelings. Emotions could relate to sympathy for a valued client or concern over not being able to medically do more for the patient. Stress of this sort is an inevitable part of the veterinary profession, and a workable plan to help veterinarians and staff manage the stress is important. A wise manager will recognize the signs of stress in the staff after an emotional farewell to a pet and not expect

Before Euthanasia is Performed

- Owner should be made aware of all alternatives.
- Owner's emotional needs and concerns are dealt with.
- Owner is educated as to the normal grief responses.
- Release form is signed by owner if this is hospital policy.
- Decision as to how to dispose of body is made.
- Financial matters are settled.
- Owner is given an opportunity to visit with the pet.
- Euthanasia procedure is explained to the owner.
- Encourage owner to bring friend or family member.

During and After Euthanasia

- Schedule procedure at as quiet a time as possible.
- Owner is given choice as to whether or not to be with pet during euthanasia.
- If owner is with pet, explain procedure and normal reactions to owner. Be sure to have facial tissue available.
- Owner is allowed to visit alone with body of pet after death. Visit should be brief and dignified. Extended visits should be discouraged.
- In cases of extreme grief, counseling should be offered, if available.
- A condolence letter or card should be sent within a few days.
- A charitable donation to an animal research fund or a veterinary college should be made in the pet's name. This is usually followed by a letter from the institution.[4]
- If the hospital is computerized and reminders for vaccinations, lab tests, etc. are sent out on an automatic basis at certain intervals, be sure that this animal is removed from that process and that the owner will not receive any such notices.

Figure 8.1 Procedures prior to and following euthanasia

"business as usual" for a reasonable period. Also to be considered is the possibility that a staff member who becomes overly involved and burdened by stress whenever an animal requires euthanasia may not be a suitable employee for an animal hospital. During your hiring interviews it is important to discuss euthanasia procedures in a limited way to determine the reaction of the prospective employee.

References

1. William F. McCulloch, DVM, MPH, *The Veterinarians Education About the Human-Animal Bond and Animal Facilitated Therapy*, *The Veterinary Clinics of North America*, Vol. 15, No. 2, March 1985, W.B. Saunders Co., p. 423
2. Jerrold Tannenbaum, MA, JD, *Veterinary Ethics*, William and Wilkins, p. 125
3. Alton F. Hopkins, DVM, "Pet Death: Affects on the Client and the Veterinarian," *The Pet Connection*, proceedings of conferences on the human-animal bond, June 13-14, 1983, the University of Minnesota, p. 278
4. Laurel S. Lagoni, Suzanne Arguello, Stephen J. Withrow, and Connee Pike, "Patient Death and Dying," *Veterinary Practice Management*, J.B. Lippincott Co., p. 315

Chapter 9

MARKETING OF VETERINARY SERVICES

What is Marketing?

"Marketing is the art and science of understanding those whose needs and wants we seek to serve, and of getting them to accept our willingness and ability to ensure their lasting satisfaction with what we provide."[1] From the standpoint of veterinary medicine, "those whose needs we seek to serve" are the owners of the animal patients that are cared for.

Veterinary medicine is a people service business. Veterinary hospitals do provide professional service to animals, but only after the agreement and support of the owner.[2] The product that is being marketed is a combination of the veterinary service itself, the place where it is being offered, and the veterinarians and staff who are providing the service. Seen in its essential elements, marketing involves communications in both directions, the hospital and the client as well as motivation of the client to seek out and purchase the services being offered. Many mistakenly consider marketing to be another nicer, more ethical, word for advertising and selling. Although marketing includes advertising and selling, it is much more. Marketing in veterinary medicine includes client relations, appearance of the hospital, listening to the owner's opinions, offering convenient practice location, providing full-service care, sending reminders, being neat and clean, sending newsletters, providing emergency service, giving career talks at high schools, using the Yellow Pages, providing handouts to clients, sending thank you notes and sympathy cards to clients, and group advertising about veterinary services. Practically everything that is done in an animal hospital in some way involves marketing. However, to be effective, there must be a serious effort on the part of management to provide planning, leadership, and controls.

Any discussion of marketing will start with a description of the "4 Ps"— product, place, price and promotion.

Product

The product of any animal hospital is the service that is provided. Services can be defined as identifiable but basically tangible activities which provide buyer satisfaction.[3] The services provided should be within the abilities of the doctors and staff to provide as well as be desired by the clientele. The service also must be professional, high quality, and people-oriented. It should be perceived and appreciated by the client as having value and be a good product.

Place

The place is obviously the hospital, clinic, automobile, or any other location where the service is provided. The place must be in a location convenient and visible to the clientele that it is meant to serve as well as be clean, neat, and attractive both inside and out. You'll need sufficient room, facilities, and equipment to provide services. You'll also need staff members who are clean, neat, personable, and who create a climate that the client will want to visit again.

Price

In a professional service business, price should not be as important an issue as it would be if your business were selling furniture or appliances. Price can, however, become a factor in areas where there are a large number of veterinarians, especially in cases of services that are either optional or can be delayed. The price that an animal hospital can charge for its services will be dependent on several factors. You will want to consider the level of knowledge that the client has about the service and the hospital and the competition in the area for that particular service. You'll need to think about the nature of the service being offered (for example, a client will be more price sensitive for a relatively routine procedure such as a vaccination), the reputation of the hospital and the veterinarians, the quality of the service, and the personal attention given to the client.

Promotion

Promotion of the services of an animal hospital involves many options. The goals of promotion should be to convince your target market of the benefits of your service, differentiate your practice from others, and build a positive practice image. Before considering the options of promotion, some definitions are in order.

- **Segmentation**—identifying a specific group of clients by specific characteristics such as age, income level, and type of pet as well as knowing which characteristics may be significant in terms of what services clients may want or what prices they are willing to pay.
- **Target marketing**—directing the promotional effort toward one or more identifiable segment.
- **Message**—what you want the client to hear.
- **Reach**—the audience reached by the message.
- **Frequency**—the average number of times that the audience is exposed to the message in a given period of time.
- **Media**—the communication channels used to send the message to the potential client.[4]

Advertising

There are several available options to promote the services of an animal hospital. The first is advertising. This is any paid form of mass communication; it is designed primarily to attract new clients to veterinary practice. Some media forms available for advertising include newspapers, magazines, television, radio, direct mail, and the Yellow Pages. There are advantages and disadvantages to each choice.

Newspapers are timely, accessible, have broad acceptance, and wide reach. The disadvantages are that this type of advertising is disposable and can be expensive, difficult to target to a specific segment, often poorly placed, and dated. Newspaper advertising is primarily suited to attract a reader who needs a product and is willing to buy it immediately.

Magazines offer superior targeting, have a long life, offer good customer acceptance, and are considered by some to be more authoritative than newspapers. The disadvantages are that it is expensive, ad placement requires a long lead time, and the effectiveness takes a long time to measure. Magazine advertising in veterinary medicine is ideally suited for group advertising such as state and national veterinary associations.

Television has wide appeal, a big reach, and frequency. Unfortunately, it is very expensive and has poor audience segmenting. Television advertising in veterinary medicine is probably only affordable in cases of group, association, or institutional advertising.

Radio has low cost, easy access, fair segmenting, and large frequency. However, there are the problems of audience inattention and little long-term impact. Radio advertising could be useful and more affordable than television for group, association, or institutional advertising.

Direct mail coupon offers are excellent for targeting and timely, and you can measure results by the response. However, there is some question as to the ethics of this option as well as the problem of junk mail perception and outdated mailing lists.

Yellow Pages may be a simple listing or a display ad. It has broad usage, long life, is a ready reference for new clients looking for an animal hospital, and can describe special or limited services. Display ads, however, are costly, and may be thought necessary only because "everyone else is doing it," not because of the return on the investment.

Any advertising should comply with the "Principles of Veterinary Medical Ethics" of the American Veterinary Medical Association (AVMA). Although the Supreme Court ruled in 1977 that professionals could advertise services, that ruling was based on the public's right to know and not to allow unfair advantage. The AVMA principles state, "A veterinarian shall not on behalf of himself, his partner, his associate, or any other veterinarian use or participate in the use of, any form of advertising or solicitation which contains a false, deceptive, or misleading statement or claim."[5] Any animal hospital advertising or contemplating advertising should refer to the AVMA's "Principles of Veterinary Medical Ethics" for more details.

Public Relations

The next promotion option to consider is public relations (PR). This is any activity initiated by your animal hospital that is designed to create a positive image while communicating with present and potential clients. Public relations allows excellent segmenting and target marketing with limited reach and frequency. There are several public relations tools available to animal hospitals.

Newsletters can be totally done in-house or purchased preprinted and personalized. They are an excellent means to educate clients about veterinary medicine in general and your hospital in particular. However, you will probably need a computerized mailing list of clients to be practical. Plus newsletters can be costly, and it may be difficult to determine their effectiveness. Newsletters are primarily a tool for internal marketing to existing clients and are directed toward retaining these clients and encouraging repeat visits.

Vaccination reminders have been part of most animal hospital procedures for many years. Reminders also are appropriate for certain laboratory examinations such as heartworm tests, dental exams, and geriatric exams. This PR tool is well accepted by clients who have come to expect them and definitely creates repeat visits. But first reminders are often not answered and a computerized reminder system is a necessity to fully use the potential. A fully utilized reminder system is the most important marketing device that any animal hospital can have. This feature alone can justify the purchase of a computer system.

Sympathy letters to clients and donations in the name of patients that have died are another effective PR tool. As noted in Chapter 8, these actions have a very positive public relations value with current clients.

Targeted letters can be sent to owners of specific patients segmented by sex, species, or age which announce new services or products as well as thank you letters for clients who refer new clients and patients. This does require a computerized client and patient list with the ability to segment.

Hospital brochures and handouts are effective marketing tools that communicate available services and products. Please see Chapter 3 for a complete discussion on what to include in a brochure.

Public appearances or talks before a service club, kennel club, school or scout group, or other similar groups are useful means to educate the public about the services available at your animal hospital. These talks can be given by the veterinarian or any knowledgeable staff member.

Special events such as hospital open houses and pet week celebrations offer opportunities to communicate and educate the public about veterinary services.

Personal Selling

The third option is known as personal selling. This is every effort made by every member of the staff to use direct personal communication, both verbal and nonverbal, to inform and persuade a client who is in the hospital or on the telephone. Examples of personal selling for the staff include personal appearance, telephone manners, listening to clients' problems, taking adequate time to explain procedures, advising clients of additional services needed for their pet, and informing clients about additional services and products available at the hospital. Personal selling also pertains to office decor and cleanliness; well-landscaped and properly maintained surroundings; signs identifying the hospital; and adequate, convenient parking.

In an established practice, the major source of continued business revenue will come from repeat business of current clients and from referrals directed to the hospital by those clients. There is no better way to create a client who becomes an ambassador for your practice than through personal selling. These clients are pleased with the service and wholeheartedly promote the practice to others. By the same taken, there is no easier way to turn a client away from the hospital and possibly create a negative voice in your midst than by poor or absent personal selling.

Publicity

Finally, there is publicity. This is any unpaid communication conveyed through the media which are newspapers, radio, or television. You can be proactively involved by mailing out press releases on local pet health issues and your own hospital news. Properly written press releases can be the basis for news stories plus position you as a news resource. Using a third party—the media—to tell your story will give it more legitimacy and credibility than will advertising.

Creating a Marketing Plan

An effective marketing plan will require many decisions that can only be made by the owners of a business. However, the manager should have some responsibility in planning something as important as a marketing plan and will certainly have a major role in the implementation of the plan. The steps in creating a marketing plan and some of the questions that have to be answered are discussed below. These steps and questions will change, depending on what stage of growth or decline that the hospital is in.

Goals

First, you and the owners must establish the mission, scope, and goals of the business. As was discussed in Chapter 1, the mission and goals of the business must be decided before anything can be accomplished. Do you want the hospital to be open 24 hours a day? Do you want to develop or employ special skills that are not being provided? Do you want to develop a business in boarding, grooming, or training? Do you want to sell pet supplies or increase food sales by nutritional counseling? Do you want to increase the number of visits per year of present clients? Do you want to attract new clients? If so, where will the new clients come from? How many hours are the veterinarians willing to work? What are the financial goals and nonfinancial goals? These and many more questions must be considered, but not necessarily answered, at this stage of planning the marketing strategy.

Market Analysis

Next, you need to analyze the market. Who are your present clients? Who are the potential new clients? Are there any new opportunities such as new housing being developed? Can the markets be segmented? Is the new housing primarily attracting elderly people or young families? Is there a means or a medium that will allow you to reach them? What services are you now providing? What new services could you provide? Are your present clients satisfied with your services? What are their problems, needs, and wants? What can you do to provide answers to their needs? Who and where is your competition? Can you differentiate your services from the competition by providing services that the competition is not or by providing a veterinary staff with board certification or specialty training? Are there any external threats such as closing of major industries, new animal hospitals, or other changes that should be considered? The primary sources for this information will be the hospital files, local news media, local chamber of commerce information, and, most importantly, client satisfaction surveys. Client surveys can yield a wealth of information to help improve client satisfaction, evaluate current offerings, test client interest in new offerings, and determine client problems, needs, and wants. They can be done in-house by sending a survey home with every client or by randomly selecting clients. Client surveys may be more effective and valuable if they can be returned to a third party. If the hospital can afford it, a survey written, distributed, and analyzed by a trained professional will give a more reliable picture of the hospital's performance and useful decision-making criteria.

Current Environment

The third step is to analyze the present situation. What are the physical facilities of the hospital? Do you have a computer to generate reminders, mailing lists, and target-market letters? What are the internal strengths of your veterinary staff, technical staff, and office staff? What are the weaknesses of your staff? Could present staff work more efficiently or possibly longer hours and see more clients? Is the hospital presently providing services which are nonproductive and should be dropped? Is the hospital and location helping or hindering long-range plans? What are the strengths and weaknesses of your equipment? What is happening to your client base? Is it growing, receding, or staying the same?

Objectives

Now you are ready to set marketing objectives. Using the information gathered from the analysis of your market and your current situation as well as your mission and goals, the next step will be to set definite objectives for the marketing plan that will include a budget to implement them. Objectives could be increasing total numbers of patients seen, seeing the same number or more patients, or increasing the number of services provided and increasing the average client dollar transaction. Objectives could be directed toward improving client relations if the client survey identified that as a problem. The objectives could be as specific as "increase number of clients seen by 25 percent" or "increase the per patient transaction by 15 percent." The objectives must be carefully considered from the standpoint of the owner's willingness to provide the time and resources to implement them.

Strategies

Now you can select the marketing strategy to implement the objectives. Will advertising be used? If so, what media will be used? Will a newsletter or target-marketing letters be used? Will a new approach to personal selling that might include hospital renovations, or new uniforms for staff be used? Will a new reminder system be installed? Will open houses be encouraged? If new services are to be added, how will you inform your present clients and prospective new clients about them?

Action Plan

Developing the action plan must be done carefully. Each strategy should be considered separately, and time and budget must be allocated for each strategy. If a newsletter, a new reminder system, or target letters are part of the strategy, does the budget include buying a computer if the hospital does not have one? If newspaper or radio advertising is to be a strategy, who will write and deliver the message, and is the budget sufficient to cover the expense. If new services, such as dental care or imaging, are to be provided, does the budget include the purchase of the equipment, the continuing education for the veterinarian and technician, and the allocation of hospital space as well as the promotion of the service to the potential client? If the strategy is to improve personal selling, the allocated budget must include the funds required for renovations and staff training.

An important part of the action plan, and often the most difficult, is to design some system to measure the results of the strategy. If the objective sets a specific goal, reaching or not reaching that goal can be the answer. Reminder systems and target letters can be measured by the return. It is not always easy to measure the results of the success of newsletters, hospital brochures, advertising, or other promotions such as open houses. Many times the only measure will be the satisfaction that the owner and staff receive from the strategy.

Plan Execution

If the mission and goals have been carefully considered, the market and the present situation analyzed, the objectives set, the marketing strategies selected, and the action plan developed, you are now ready to execute the plan. The key issues here will be to contract for the services of the consultants, advertisers, and other needed vendors as well as purchasing the necessary equipment and learning how to use it. You'll need to schedule the promotions, manage the allocated budget, and measure the results.[6]

A marketing plan does not have to be a long, time-consuming process to be effective. The important considerations are

- What is it that you want to be?
- What situations surround you?
- What are you now?
- What do you have to do to get from where you are to where you want to be?
- How do you do it?

Marketing and the Computer

If most of the computers currently in use in animal hospitals today are given information on the client (such as name, address, and occupation) and information on the patients (such as breed, sex, age, and vaccination and medical history), the computer can provide effective marketing tools.

- **Reminders** for any vaccination or medical procedure provided by the hospital. The computer can be programmed to automatically provide these reminders for all patients requiring the service at predetermined intervals. Individual clients also can be programmed to receive future reminders for any service or inventory item. The computer also will tell you if the reminder has been answered by the client and, if not, provide an unlimited number of repeat reminders. The reminders can be personalized and printed in letter form, on specially designed postcards, or on callback lists. Postal permits can be programmed into the computer printing and the reminders can be generated and processed by zip codes which greatly reduces mailing expense.
- **Callback lists** as reminders to staff to check on the progress of a patient or remind a client of an appointment.
- **Target letters** for certain species, diseases, ages, and practice areas can be written and merged with names and addresses of clients owning those animals or living in those areas. For example, you could decide to send a letter to all clients owning animals over eight years of age, suggesting a geriatric workup; letters to all cat owners suggesting a new vaccine; or letters to all people living in two specific zip code areas warning about a heartworm outbreak. Those letters could be personalized with both the owner's and the pet's names. The work involved on your part would be to write the letter once and tell the computer the characteristics for whom the letter was to be sent.
- **Mailing lists** of all the hospital's clients or certain clients, such as those who have been to the hospital in the last year, or those who have not been there in the last year, or those who have spent $100.00 or more. These lists could be printed onto envelopes or mailing labels and used for mass printings such as newsletters.
- **Prewritten messages and reminders** on receipts that are sent home with the client after a hospital visit that will help the client better understand the provided services and the reasons for the charges.[7]

An intangible benefit from a computer is that if the computer is well programmed and competently operated, the hospital will be well run, efficient, and give a sense of satisfaction to the client. Today's clients respect what a computer can do and know that if the hospital is using a computer, then it is providing a high-quality service. The computer will be another example that the animal hospital you are managing understands the needs and wants of those it seeks to serve and is doing its best.

References

1. Francis G. Edwards, *Marketing of Professional Services*, Pennwell Publishing Co., p. 35
2. Dennis M. McCurnin, DVM, *Veterinary Practice Management*, J.B. Lippincott Co., p. 116
3. American Veterinary Medical Association, *Marketing and Practice Strategies*, July 1988, p. 3
4. James F. Engel, Martin R. Warshaw, Thomas C. Kinnear, *Promotional Strategy - Managing the Marketing Communications Process*, Irwin, 1987, Chapters 5 and 15
5. American Veterinary Medical Association, *Principles of Veterinary Medical Ethics*, 1988 AVMA Directory, p. 452
6. Margo Murray-Hicks, "Marketing Basics for Small Entrepreneurs," lecture presented at Training 88 Conference, December 14, 1988, Margo Murray-Hicks and Assoc., Oakland, Calif.
7. Owen E. McCafferty, CPA, "Computers: Luxury or Necessity?" *Veterinary Economics*, March 1989, p. 67

Chapter 10

COMPUTER USE

by Robert H. Featherston, DVM, MS

Computers can be used to enhance the performance of almost all the management activities described in previous chapters. This chapter will address what to consider when you plan, select, and install a computer system, regardless of whether it is your first computer or an upgrade of a current system in your practice.

Before you computerize, it is important that you first review the overall needs of your veterinary practice. Avoid the temptation to make even a tentative selection of specific hardware and software until you complete an analysis, similar to that outlined in this chapter, of your own hospital functions. Your ultimate objective is to develop an effective, automated information processing system for your practice—not just to install a computer system.

Since a computerized hospital information system is a significant investment, part of your overall plan must include staff training and ongoing management control. In order to achieve a good return on your investment, these elements are crucial.

Computer Use by Veterinarians is Growing

While few veterinarians were using computers in their practices in the 1970s[1], by the end of the 1980s, automation systems in veterinary practices accelerated. In January of 1992, the American Veterinary Medical Association conducted a survey to determine the extent of computer usage in private clinical practice.[2] The survey revealed that computers were used in 58% of the practices. Among veterinarians using computers, software specifically designed for veterinary practice management was used most often—by 86% of small animal-exclusive practitioners and 77% of all private clinical practitioners.

Analysis also showed a clear relationship between computer use and the number of veterinarians participating in a single clinic. Computers were in use in 43% of the single-veterinarian clinics. However, computers were in use in 60% of the three-veterinarian practices, and in 80% of the four-or-more-veterinarian practices.

But if this survey were completed today, the level of computer use by veterinarians would be higher since the cost of hardware and specialized software has significantly decreased. Even those veterinary clinics with only one or two practitioners are now finding automated systems affordable. Cost reductions also are enabling practitioners who have been relying on older systems to upgrade to larger, faster, and more efficient systems. As more veterinarians take advantage of the improving technology, those who continue to manage their operations with manual systems will find themselves at a competitive disadvantage.

There are a variety of reasons to automate. From a business standpoint, automation can reduce costs, produce more timely reporting of critical information, increase marketing capabilities, and efficiently restructure staff operations. From a professional standpoint, it can lead to improved patient care and endow your clinic with additional prestige while you stay on top of operations at your practice.

If you are thinking of automating or upgrading, it will be helpful to keep these advantages in mind. Installation of an automated system is a significant capital investment and requires ongoing attention to system management. It also requires a sense of commitment. The rewards, however, can be both significant and numerous.

When considering a new or upgraded information system, most veterinarians begin by speculating about what the system might do for their practice. Even if they perceive certain advantages, they then find themselves agonizing over the question of whether the system will warrant the investment. Therefore, the first step in the automation decision-making process is to review and document in detail the tasks that you presently perform in your own practice and the systems you use to handle these tasks. The remainder of this chapter will outline a procedure to help you determine if automation is appropriate for your practice.

Elements of the Analysis Process

In their book, *Computers in Private Practice*[3], Byron Oberst and John Long recommend that medical practitioners begin the process of determining what, if anything, they should do about automating by taking a careful look at six aspects of their practice. Their suggestions to physicians are equally appropriate for veterinarians. They recommend that you examine the following subjects:

- **Current systems**—Identify the information-generating systems you use in your practice today, including your manual systems. Define the way you do things now and pay particular attention to activities in which there is duplication of effort.
- **Problem areas**—Is the number of transactions in your practice leveling off? Are your expenses increasing? Does the rate of staff turnover concern you? Pinpoint and detail

problem areas, including those that may not appear directly related to management information procedures.

- **Priorities**—What are the most urgent problems that confront you in your practice? Patient invoicing? Low client retention rate? Is response rate to patient-care reminders below industry standards? Inventory control? Lack of timely financial information? Personal stress? After you identify your problems, try to rank them in declining order of severity.
- **Alternatives**—Make a candid analysis of what you might do in an attempt to deal with the problems and priorities you have identified. One alternative, of course, is to do nothing.
- **Relative Costs**—Start to develop realistic cost figures if you conclude that a new or upgraded computer system is a viable alternative. Operational savings resulting from computerization also should be considered. Keep in mind that these savings may be both direct and indirect. Careful analysis of operational savings and profit improvement will allow you to calculate the cost benefit for the optional computer systems under consideration.[4]
- **Projected Plan**—Be realistic when you detail the alternative you identify as your most intelligent option.

As you prepare to undertake this analysis, it is important that your staff members be candidly advised of your intention to evaluate your present system and, possibly, replace it. They also should be reassured. If you choose to computerize, make it clear to your staff that their positions are not in jeopardy. Emphasize that automation of your information functions has the potential to make their work less frustrating and more interesting. Solicit their help in your analytical study.

Analyze Your Current System

The first step in determining what changes, if any, need to be made in your office information procedures is to make a careful analysis of the procedures you use now. Such an analysis is important, as it would be counter-productive to move to a new computer system if your current manual systems don't make sense. For example, if your accounts receivable process is not working well now, its not going to suddenly work better when you put the same data in a computer.

Along with a review and description of all your manual operations, prepare a description of how you would like these operations to be performed if they were placed under computer control. Software programs can be accurately prescribed only if there is a clear understanding of the results the programs are expected to produce. This step is extremely important and should not be overlooked.

Moreover, you should be aware that even the most talented computer consultant cannot help you evaluate software programs unless you provide a clear understanding of current operations and the results you would like to achieve. If your present information system has problems, it also is important to determine if these problems are caused by inadequacies in the system or by its ineffective use.

Intelligent analysis of your current system requires that you do more than take a surface look at your operation. Dig deep. Find out how your information system actually works—or doesn't work.

When you conduct an analysis of your present system, focus your attention on the following key areas:

- **Business data**

  Daily activity reports and control procedures
  Accounts receivable
  Accounts payable
  Practice analysis reports
  Payroll
  Inventory control
  General ledger
  Record security

- **Practice management**

  Patient admission and release procedures
  Immunization compliance rate
  Recall and recheck system effectiveness
  Scheduling of appointments
  No-show follow up
  Client retention rate
  Patients medical records
  Record security

- **Professional and marketing applications**

  Word processing for professional and marketing communications
  Development of client educational and instruction materials

- **Reference access**

Access to national databases and communication with other practitioners through services such as the National Libraries of Medicine (MEDLINE) and the Network of Animal Health (NOAH).

In the process of making a detailed analysis of your current system, there are critical considerations to help you determine whether the system functions efficiently. Ask yourself the following questions:

- **Personnel**—Is your staff well trained in the use of the current system? Is the staff capable of using the system effectively? Do responsible staff members actually understand what the present system is designed to do?
- **Accuracy of the system**—How confidently do you rely on data now being produced in your practice?
- **Degree of duplication in data entry**—Are there situations in your routine operations where the same information is typed or written as many as four or five times?
- **Quality and consistency of results**—When confronted with the same type of practice problem, do different staff members follow the same procedures and achieve the desired results?
- **Data volume and flow**—Does your system produce accurate, timely information from which you or other professionals in your practice can make intelligent decisions? Good computerized systems for veterinary hospitals display on-screen menus that have the effect of forcing staff members to follow the forms and enter all required information.
- **Patient flow**—Does your current system allow you and your staff to confidently make and keep client appointments, sparing clients the annoyance of time-consuming delays before proceeding to the examination room?
- **Security controls**—Does your current system include built-in controls to protect against inaccurate data entry in patient and financial records?
- **Cost of operation**—In addition to analyzing the effectiveness and accuracy of your current information system, make a realistic attempt to determine its cost. Manual systems often require more staff time than do automated systems that produce the same results. You need to be able to make an objective comparison of such costs.

Identify Problem Areas

Identification of problem areas in your practice is an important element when analyzing your current information system. Try to pinpoint all operating results that you consider to be problems, not just those that appear to be directly connected with your current information system. For example, if you detect a measurable decline in your active client base, you should identify that as a problem area in your practice. But could such a decline be attributed to a shortcoming in your existing information system? Careful analysis might show a relationship between the two. In any event, you should make an objective effort to identify all existing problem areas in your practice. The following are some of the symptoms to watch for in your analysis:

- high level of accounts receivable
- inability to collect fees at the time of treatment
- decline in or leveling off of net income
- increase in practice expenses
- decline in productivity (more staff required to produce same results)
- high staff turnover
- excessive volume of paperwork
- high level of stress, both in staff and veterinarians
- inability to keep on projected daily schedule
- decline in patient load
- excessive down time (too many open appointment slots)
- decrease in immunization compliance
- low number of per year visits by individual patients
- decrease in active client base
- low inventory turnover rate and/or high shrinkage

In addition, a number of benchmarks provide some indication as to the financial health of a veterinary practice. Not all, of course, equally apply to every practice. Moreover, the degree of importance of a particular problem tends to be relative rather than absolute. The following are typical potential problems in a veterinary hospital which may signal the need for attention:[5]

- **Disappointing revenue growth**—Compare your revenue growth today with growth in previous quarters or years, and compare it with the growth of the economy as a whole. Make due allowance for inflation.
- **Erosion of profit**—Compare your recent profit figures with earlier profit yields during similar periods. Also compare your profit results with profit projections you have made, and with published profit ratios for the veterinary profession.
- **Internal factors suggesting a less-than-desirable financial operation**—Look for negative factors such as an increase in bad debt losses, growing overtime costs, inven-

tory shrinkage, reduced inventory turnover, lengthening of the average age of receivables, reduced revenue per veterinarian, and similar indications.

- **Hectic work environment**—Seek to make a candid appraisal of such factors as general disorder, staff errors, staff omissions, high staff turnover, and a work environment characterized by staff members lurching from problem to problem.
- **Absence of basic information**—Evaluate whether you are able to routinely determine how actual hospital operations relate to your planned budget and whether you are able to detect early signs of adverse trends in revenues, client base, and productivity.
- **Lack of uniformity in hospital information**—Does the quality and completeness of data entered in your basic hospital records vary widely from patient to patient? If so, be aware that on-screen displays of patient information forms in software designed for veterinary hospitals prompts entry of complete, uniform data on each client/patient transaction.

As you conduct this analysis of your practice and installation of a computer system appears to be logical, estimates as to the size of the system needed will be controlled by the figures you collect. Most vendors of veterinary computer systems can provide detailed work sheets that relate system size to numbers connected with a specific practice. Figures you compile should include accurate estimates as to the number of

- client/patient records
- new patients per year
- patient visits per year
- transactions per year
- accounts receivable
- staff and job designations
- number of work areas
- number of inventory items

In addition, your compilation should include data that describes the aging of past-due accounts, the amount of bookkeeping done in-house, and the scope of medical records you desire to maintain. With this type of information available, vendors with whom you discuss optional automated systems will be in a much better position to define which systems are appropriate for your practice.

Establish Objectives and Priorities

After you complete the analysis of your current information processing system, you will be ready to define your new objectives. If you perceive shortcomings in your current system, you will be in a better position to identify your objectives in each area of your practice. You can thus compare your new objectives with current results. This exercise will help you better understand what you need to do to reach the defined objectives. It also will help you establish goals that are realistic for your particular practice.

No two veterinarians will establish the same objectives for their individual information processing systems. Emphasis will vary from practice to practice, and objectives that have a high priority in one practice will have a lower priority in another.

The following are general objectives for you to consider as you plan for an improved information processing system:

- **Client account data readily available on demand.** Ideally, up-to-date account data for each individual client should be available at all times for immediate printout or on-screen viewing. When you review the status of a client's account, it should not be necessary to stop and construct the account data from a variety of sources.

- **Current staff will have little or no difficulty using the system.** No matter how appealing an otherwise desirable information system might appear, it is not worth considering if its implementation will require replacement of your clinic staff. An improved information system should be viewed as a helpful support device for you and your personnel, not as a hindrance. A primary purpose in improving your information processing system is to improve efficiency without creating additional operating costs. A system which requires that you add more people in order to operate the system negates this purpose.

- **Access to management data on demand.** To efficiently manage a modern veterinary clinic, you must have access to current, accurate data on all aspects of the operation—on everything from the status of inventory stocks to overdue accounts. Your system should be designed to quickly provide you with the precise information you need. Furthermore, access to the information should require nothing more than typing in a few letters or numbers on the keyboard.

- **Generate meaningful management reports.** To make the "right" decisions in a veterinary clinic, the professional in charge must make decisions based on accurate, easy-to-understand information. However, veterinary practitioners are often compelled to base their decisions on data from outside accountants or consultants—data which is difficult to comprehend. Ideally, an information processing system in a veterinary clinic should produce reports which are clear and meaningful.

- **A system that produces a complete audit trail.** Even in the best information systems, occasional errors will intrude. For example, a charge for services not performed will appear on a client's invoice. In such instances, it is important that the system allow the practitioner to identify the *source* of the error. Unfortunately, in some clinics, computer-generated data is treated as omnipotent. (i.e. "It must be right if its in the computer.") Insist that the system installed in your clinic allows you to quickly track down the source of any data subject to question.

- **Reduce duplication and paperwork.** A decade ago, it was commonplace for different staff members in a veterinary clinic to write a client's name more than a dozen times in connection with a single visit. The first entry was made when the appointment was recorded; the final entry was made when the client was billed. Between these two events, the name of the client (or patient) was recorded in a variety of other records, logs, and orders. Not only is this exercise repetitive, but also it's a time-waster and an invitation to error. Strive for an information system that eliminates, as much as possible, duplication of data entry.

- **A system that provides security for your records in event of a fire or employee embezzlement.** Client/patient records that accumulate over the years come to constitute the very foundation of a veterinary practice. The practitioner who does not have access to patient records is, in a sense, starting from ground zero each time he sees a long-time patient. Unfortunately, a fire or other natural catastrophe can destroy these records in an instant. There also are situations in which staff may deliberately destroy, remove, or alter pre-existing records. To protect your practice from such devastating events, your information system should include a feature which routinely duplicates records on a backup system such as tapes or a removable hard-drive cartridge system. These duplicate records can then be transferred periodically to a secure, off-site location such as a safe deposit box.

Establish Application Priorities for Your System

As explained previously, the first step toward improvement of the information procedures in your practice is to make an in-depth analysis of the current procedures. Second, establish objectives for improvement of the system. By establishing objectives, you can better visualize what features appear to be essential in a new system.

With your objectives in mind, the next step is to develop a list of priorities. Reaching select, defined objectives will be more critical than reaching others. Once you identify special priorities in your practice, you and your vendors will be better able to assess the needs and identify the type of system that fits your practice.

What priorities might you deem important in your clinic? Here are some possibilities.

- **More detailed patient invoicing and accounts receivable records**—Your analysis may reveal that patient invoices should include data not presently displayed, and that your accounts receivable records should provide a more detailed picture of these accounts.

- **Productivity reports**—Do your present records reveal the relationship between the professional staff and the fees generated? If not, it may be a priority for your practice to generate individual productivity reports.
- **Word processing that will merge with client/patient databases**—There are situations in all veterinary practices in which the same type of "personalized" information needs to be sent to select clients. However, if a separate notice is prepared for each client, the word processing time involved can be prohibitive. Fortunately, modern veterinary software systems permit the staff to prepare a single message and then print out a personal message to multiple clients.
- **Easy-to-use search and sort capability**—If you need information on a particular patient, does someone in your office shuffle through scores of files? If you need to identify a particular segment of your clients or patients, must the job be done by hand? If so, you probably need to consider a system that includes search and sort capability.
- **Inventory control**—Your investment in pharmaceuticals, medical supplies, and patient diets represents a substantial portion of your operating expenses. If your current system does not provide reorder information, discount levels, and similar details on the status of this inventory, installation of a system that will produce such information could be a priority requirement for your practice.
- **General ledger**—Is your financial information available on a timely basis? Does your basic bookkeeping tool, the ledger, presently generate the information you need for effective management? For tax records? For investment decisions? If not, the need for a more efficient system may be indicated.
- **Payroll**—Does your payroll system automatically calculate deductions, taxes, and other data for each employee? Or, are these functions still performed manually?
- **Reminder and recall system**—Is someone in your clinic alert enough to remember when it's time to notify a particular client of immunization schedules? Or is this information generated automatically? If you are still relying on someone's memory and a manual system and you have difficulty tracking client response rate, a system that will handle these functions should probably get a high priority in your planning.
- **Medical records**—In a discussion with a client, are you able to bring up a computer screen which details records regarding a particular patient? Or must you rifle through a pile of papers in hope of finding and being able to read the records? A system that would instantly generate accurate and legible records would save time and money and also would enhance the prestige of your practice.
- **Spreadsheet capabilities**—A veterinary practice is a professional venture and thereby entails all the characteristics of any business—including the potential for profit and loss. Today, no top-level executive would think of attempting to manage without having spreadsheets available reflecting details of the operation: budgeting, cash flow, av-

erage transactions, inventory investment, etc. Spreadsheets can be of enormous value in making management decisions, particularly if they are coupled with charts that graphically display trends in the business.

In your practice, there may be other objectives to which you assign a higher priority. The rationale behind the analytic approach is to help you identify on a methodical, step-by-step basis the characteristics of the information system that best meets the needs of your individual practice.

Alternatives Available for Your Decision Making

After you have completed an analysis of your present information system and have established a set of objectives and priorities for the system you might want to install, you will need to make one of the following decisions:

- **Do nothing**. Deciding to stay with your current system with no changes of any kind is a decision in itself.
- **Train or hire staff to use your current system more effectively**. You may determine that your present system meets your needs but is not being used in the manner in which it was designed to be used. Such a conclusion may dictate retraining current staff or possibly hiring additional staff to make the system work. In some practices this might necessitate the hiring of an office manager or hospital administrator.
- **Select a computerized system**. If you decide to select a new system, then you will be confronted with additional analysis requirements which are outlined in more detail below.
- **Upgrade to a more advanced computer system**. Select software enhancements together with hardware that provides greater storage capacity and faster operating speed.

If you select either the third or fourth of these alternatives, you will need to proceed further with your analysis-and-decision process, and specifically with the cost analysis process. If you are going to use a computer system for the first time, or you are going to upgrade your current computer system, you will need to make a general determination as to what the move will cost. A useful reference for this determination is Dr. James W. Allens, *Hospital Computer Systems for Health Professionals: A Cost-Benefit Approach to Assessing Alternative Technologies*.[6]

In analyzing costs involved in a move to computerization, you need to consider two aspects of a computer system: acquisition costs and recurring costs. The principal items to consider relative to your initial costs (or acquisition costs) include

- computer hardware and software costs;
- costs to prepare your hospital site for computerization: cable installation, electrical wiring, environmental controls, etc.;
- initial training of your personnel, both on-site and off-site, in use of the new system;
- actual installation costs (hardware installation and software configuration);
- time costs, both for the staff and the veterinarian to enter client/patient data into the new system;
- costs to create a computer "environment"—remodeling of desks, counters, and cabinets to accommodate equipment; printer stands;
- supplies: toner, disks, backup tapes, paper, printer ribbons, printed letterheads, and postcards.

In addition, the system will involve several recurring costs.

- Maintenance and support services provided by outside consultants and service firms.
- Costs to retrain staff at intervals as personnel changes and software programs are added or upgraded.
- Cost of eventually upgrading the system (the typical efficient life of a computer system is from four to seven years).

A well-designed information system will allow staff members to redirect their activities toward patient care and client relations and away from paperwork. It also will improve the accuracy of your financial operations and enhance your marketing efforts. But, one of the most important benefits of a good system is reduction in stress throughout the hospital staff.

Although some of the benefits of an advanced computer system are intangible, each adds value to the operation of a veterinary hospital. In evaluating the cost/benefit ratio of an automated system, do not overlook the value provided by such hard-to-measure benefits as improved staff morale, reduction in paperwork, or enhanced client relations.

When estimating the initial cost of your projected system, evaluate the cost of hardware and software separately. The cost of software will vary from vendor to vendor. Some vendors will sell only a complete software package while others will sell application modules to fit specific needs. The cost of software will vary according to such factors as

- required applications
- additional programming costs
- staff training
- vendor support

Hardware costs are dependent upon factors such as current and projected storage volume that may be required to use the system, speed of operation, and whether workstations will need to be connected through a network which is controlled by special software. Peripheral requirements (number of workstations, number and types of printers, fax or modem connections, etc.) also influence the cost of hardware. In addition, hardware costs depend on the vendor you select and the amount of technical support you expect from the vendor.

Dealing with Vendors

In many small businesses, it makes sense for the owner to create a computer system simply by purchasing off-the-shelf hardware and software from an electronics store. However, in the veterinary practice, this approach does not work. Veterinary hospitals need systems in which there is complete integration between the databases created for each phase of the operation: patient records, client records, inventory records, and billing records. Certain entries made in patient records, for example, should be simultaneously and automatically interfaced with the client records without having to physically key in the information.

Because of this need for a "seamless" system to integrate data from each venue of the hospital, companies which specialize in computerized systems for veterinary practices have emerged in the marketplace. There are a number of such vendor firms now active, and each offers a somewhat different configuration of hardware, software, and support services.

When you find yourself evaluating a new computer system, it is useful to consult with at least two—preferably more—of these vendors during the initial stages of your investigation. You need to get a feel for the package of services offered by each. It also helps to ask the vendor about the level of technical support you might expect to receive. It is critical when you make your final decision that you select the "right" vendor for your practice.

Purchase of a veterinary hospital computer system is not like the purchase of a commodity. The transaction does not end when the product is delivered. Rather, the purchase of your computer system should mark the beginning of a close, ongoing relationship between you and the vendor. Following the purchase, you will need to look to the vendor for help with technical problems, staff training, and system upgrades as computer technology advances. For this reason, it is important to select a vendor with whom you are comfortable and in whom you have confidence.

As you evaluate potential vendors and proceed toward your ultimate purchase decision, keep in mind these guidelines.[7]

- Be sure to purchase from an established vendor. You need to make sure the vendor will still be around when you need help.

- Review the vendor's financial status. If the supplier is a closely held or private company, review the financial stability of its principals.
- Make your initial purchase of all hardware and software from the same vendor and have it all covered under a single maintenance agreement. If a problem arises, this arrangement will eliminate disputes as to whether the problem is software- or hardware-related.
- Strive to negotiate a contract which calls for the vendor to respond within four hours or less when you need technical support.
- To prevent misunderstandings, get all promises from vendors in writing. Document your discussions with vendor representatives by sending memos to their companies in which you outline your understanding of what the representative has promised. Ask for verification in writing.
- Don't neglect to review space and environmental requirements that will be created by your system—especially electrical surge control protection.
- Adequately insure your system through a policy obtained from an agent who is knowledgeable about computers.

Similar precautions should be taken when you purchase software for your system. Keep in mind these points when you make your final decision on purchasing software.

- Have each prospective software vendor give you a written statement that explains where the vendor's software codes can be obtained in the event of default or bankruptcy on the part of the vendor.
- Arrange for an attorney knowledgeable in computer contracts to review your projected contract documents and to prepare points for clarification. Do not sign until these points have been clarified to your satisfaction.
- Try to keep two vendors under consideration until your final software purchase decision is made.

Prior to the purchase of software, try to verify that both the vendor and the software programs have good track records, particularly in the veterinary hospital market. Ask for a list of users of the programs. Check with some of them to see if they are satisfied with the support they have received from the vendor, and if there has been a good history of program improvements or updates.

It is important that you receive a detailed demonstration of the program and that you make a site visit to an installed system. Do not make a decision based on a demonstration of a system without assurance that the demonstration was based on the use of a large database of clients and patients. (The amount of time required for the performance of a software function can be drastically affected by the amount of data to be accessed and searched.)

In your final evaluation of systems under consideration, involve as many of your hospital staff as possible in the process. Arrange for staff who perform special functions to attempt these same functions on each of the systems under consideration. Develop a rating procedure to facilitate an objective analysis and comparison of the systems under consideration. Here are some of the functions that should be carefully compared.

- The number of keystrokes required and the menu screen changes for given functions.
- Review output reports and the ability to modify report formats.
- File-sorting and running-time estimates for the major applications of the system.
- Backup procedures, including the amount of time required for backups and the optimum interval between each backup.
- Purging procedures for old files.
- Clarity and readability of the user manuals for the software under consideration. Is a level of education beyond a high school degree required for an understanding of the instructions? Do the help screens in the software programs provide adequate information, or will additional training be required?

Planning and Implementation

At this point, you may have completed the analysis process and identified the special needs in your practice for a new or upgraded computer system. You may have even selected a system vendor. Does this mean your involvement with implementing a new system has finally ended? Not quite. Although your vendor will handle most of the technical details required to get the system installed and running efficiently, you also must address the following issues:

- **Training your staff in operation of the system.** No matter how technically advanced your new system may be, it will not work well until your staff members are comfortable with it.
- **Determining which services should be included and omitted in your systems database.** One of the advantages of computerized systems in a veterinary hospital is that staff employees need enter only a three- or four-digit code in a patient's record to identify a medical service provided for that patient. However, the generic list of such services included in your software selection can be extensive. You need to determine if the list includes services that do not apply to your practice or if the list omits services which your practice offers.

- **Determining when to enter data.** You may decide to gradually key your current patient information into the new system over an extended period of six months to a year. The other option is to enter all details as quickly as possible.[8]

A carefully thought-out decision on each of these issues will be essential to the overall success of your new computer system. While your vendor should have extensive experience installing similar systems in other veterinary hospitals, your thorough understanding of the details of your own practice necessitates your active participation in the transition process. As you make the transition, there are several points to keep in mind.

Staff Training

When planning the installation and implementation of a new system, make sure you allow ample time for staff training. The actual installation of the system should be scheduled to occur during a relatively slow time in your practice.

Do not rely on the hope that staff members will "catch on" to the new system after it has been in operation for awhile. In your contract, state that the vendor should conduct training sessions during the transition period. If your staff has confidence in the operation of the system, your hospital will benefit from more efficient operations.

Selection of Database Fields

All computer systems designed for veterinary hospitals include predefined patient and client databases. These databases contain extensive lists of typical services and activities connected with veterinary practice. Each service or activity field is assigned a three- or four-digit code. For example, under the heading, "Outpatient Services," a patient database offered by a vendor, basic and specific fields might include

100 — Office Visit/Examination
101 — Emergency Office Visit
102 — Puppy Examination
103 — Comprehensive Examination

Further into the database the fields become more specific. For instance

121 — Examination with DHLPP Puppy Vaccine
128 — Examination with FVRCP Annual Vaccine
138 — Examination with Parvovirus Vaccine

Adjacent to each of these database fields, there is a place to enter the fee charged for that specific service. The system also is configured to enter other coded information with each database entry.

The databases offered by vendors to veterinary hospitals also include similar coded fields for pharmaceuticals, vaccines, and surgical supplies such as

791 — Metronidazole Tablets 250mg
313 — Dist-Hep-Parainflu Vac. (3 wk)
4731 — Orthopedic Surgical Pack

Once the system is in operation, staff members will need to enter only one or two code numbers in a patient's computer file for services rendered. The system itself will follow through with all other necessary information entries such as tax computation, client billing, follow-up reminders, and medical reference. For this reason, the information encrypted into the database is of utmost importance, as it controls all other data generated by the system.

Since vendors who specialize in computer systems for veterinarians have extensive experience with a variety of veterinary clinics, their generic databases include coded fields for almost every conceivable service, product, or activity that might be available from a veterinary practice. Although the databases for veterinary practices are extensive and accurate, they are not universally appropriate for all veterinarians.

Pay close attention to each coded field. Determine if the described field is pertinent to your practice, and delete those fields which are not. Add fields for services offered in your practice that do not appear in the vendor's generic database.

When you conduct this review exercise, it is useful to confer with other veterinary practitioners who have adopted the same system. Request copies of the databases they are using. Seek their counsel as to services that should be deleted from or added to the basic coded fields of services. Also, request copies of their report formats which are generated from information in the database.

A line-by-line analysis of the database also helps to solicit input from your staff. Get their opinion as to which service fields should be included and which should not. As a rule, it is better to start out with too few fields than with too many. It also is much easier to define these coded fields at the onset than to change them at a later date. If you decide to add or delete items after the system has been in operation for a year or two, information produced by the system will lack historical consistency.

Configure the database for your new system to conform with your perception of what it should contain. For example, if you rely on a defined chart of financial accounts and it serves your practice well, there is no reason not to transfer the same account categories into your new system. By doing so, you will be able to continue making valid comparisons with earlier financial results. Both you and your accountant will tend to be more comfortable with the system. In addition, you will save time that would otherwise be spent structuring new financial procedures to conform with earlier ones.

Entering Data Into Your New System

No matter how well configured your new computerized system may be, it will be totally useless without data. The system will be incapable of searching a patient's records until those records have first been entered into the system.

Once your system has been installed, and after you and your staff have selected the coded data fields, you will need to enter the hard data on your patients, clients, financial operations, and other aspects of your practice. As stated earlier, you have two options for entering your data—all information immediately, or gradually with current active clients.

What are the advantages to enter all client/patient data into your system after installation? First, your staff will become familiar and comfortable with how the system operates. Next, once the database is complete, their clerical workload will be reduced since it will only be necessary to update information on active and new clients and patients.

Immediate creation of the client/patient database also permits immediate use of the database for current reminders and marketing activities. The sooner your database is completed, the sooner your practice can begin to reap the benefits of computerization.

The most obvious disadvantage to inputting information upon installation is that it imposes a heavy workload on your staff. It will be next to impossible for your staff to take on this assignment while continuing with their routine duties. This means it will be necessary to hire temporary employees whose sole duty is to enter data into your new system. Another disadvantage is that the computer database you create only will be as accurate as your previous record system. Temporary employees will not be able to identify outdated or inaccurate information; they will simply enter it into the new system.

The alternative approach is to identify a group of clients who are currently active clients and to gradually enter basic information only on these clients. A second group also might be chosen for entry, which would consist of clients destined to receive reminders from your office in the months immediately ahead.

The chief advantage of the gradual approach is that the keying of information can be handled by your own staff. In addition, the data that is entered tends to be both current and accurate since out-of-date phone numbers, addresses, and details on patient status are less likely to end up in the database when information is gradually entered.

The disadvantage is that it will take at least a year to get the majority of your clients entered into the system. During this period, your staff must rely on a parallel manual reminder system to ensure that timely notices are sent to all clients. During this period, you also will not have the benefits of a complete database. For example, you will not be able to conduct reliable search and sort activities.

However you choose to enter information in your database, it is recommended that you give first priority to entering data on clients with accounts receivable. By doing so, you will be able to maintain efficient billing and aging cycles. On the other hand, it is not recommended that you initially enter detailed medical information for all clients. Usually, basic information related to the client, patient, and reminder notices will be sufficient. Medical information can be added once your primary records are in place.

Even if you choose to bring in temporary help to enter data, your permanent staff also should be given responsibility to enter some data. This participation will give them an understanding of the available coded fields in your database. They also will become more familiar with the fields and will better grasp the type of information that should be collected and entered for both clients and patients. Staff members will ultimately develop a better understanding of the system.

Other Considerations During the Implementation Period

After you have entered a reasonable amount of data into your new system, a review of reports the system can generate is in order. You should test the system to make sure it is capable of displaying or printing the reports you need in the most useful form.

It helps to begin generating these reports while the vendor is at your practice. The vendor can assist in formatting the reports in a style that best serves the needs of you and your staff as well as the needs of your clients. It is helpful to experiment with a variety of different report formats before establishing which ones to use on a permanent basis.

Also, during the implementation period, you should develop the text of client messages you wish to keep stored in your computer system. Such messages might include vaccine reminder notices, delinquent account notices, marketing letters, and client education documents. After writing these messages, they can be printed out on a personalized basis at any time.

If you use preprinted letterheads, invoices, statements, and similar forms, seek help from your vendor representative in the layout and formatting of such documents.

During the implementation stage, it is advisable to establish staff responsibilities for various aspects of the system's operation. For example, assign the responsibility to back up computer records on a regular basis. In addition, someone must take responsibility to order computer supplies and arrange for routine system maintenance. Also, various staff must be assigned the responsibility to enter specific data on a regular basis.

In summary, follow these progressive steps when moving your practice into a new or advanced computer system:

- Make a detailed analysis of all aspects of your practice and identify problem areas.
- Establish clear objectives for the information system you believe you would like to install in your practice. Classify these objectives in order of declining priority.
- Evaluate vendors of computer systems designed specifically for veterinary hospitals. Investigate the background and reliability of the vendor or vendors whom you feel can best serve your needs.

- After selecting a vendor, carefully review the coded fields in the vendor's standard database. Revise or delete fields as necessary to make them conform to the needs of your own practice.
- Decide whether to enter data into your new system on a gradual or immediate basis.

The procedures outlined in this chapter may strike you as being laborious and time-consuming. Remember, though, that your hospital information system serves, in effect, as both the neurological network and the heart of your practice. The system plays a critical role in every aspect of your day-to-day operations. That is why it is important that you devote adequate time and careful attention to an analysis of your practice before you proceed to the selection of a new information system. The rewards will be substantial. Selection of the right system from the right vendor will produce more tightly focused management control, smoother operations, a happier staff, and clear cost benefits—in other words, a greatly improved professional environment for your practice.

References

1. Phillip L. Farber, "History of Computers in Veterinary Practice," *The Veterinary Clinics of North America*, July 1986, p. 609-614
2. J. Karl Wise, PhD, Jih-Jing, PhD, "Computer Use and Applications in Veterinary Medicine," *Journal of the American Veterinary Medical Association*, 1992; 201:1352-1354
3. Byron B. Oberst, John M. Long, *Computers in Private Practice Management*, Springer-Verlag, 1987, Chapter 13
4. David P. Gallagher, MA, "Economic and Management Considerations of a Computer," *The Veterinary Clinics of North America*, July 1986, p. 729-743
5. Donald R. Shaw, *Your Small Business Computer: Evaluating, Selecting, Financing, Installing and Operating Hardware and Software That Fits*, Van Nostrand Reinhold Co., 1981, Chapter 9
6. James W. Allen, MD, MS, *Hospital Computer Systems for Health Professionals: A Cost-Benefit Approach to Assessing Alternative Technologies*, McGraw-Hill, Inc. 1990, Chapter 6
7. John P. Sheridan, Owen E. McCafferty, *The Business of Veterinary Practice*, Pergamon Press, 1993, p. 104-105
8. David H. Taylor, "Effects of Computers on the Practice," *The Veterinary Clinics of North America*, July 1986, p. 713-715

Appendix A

MANAGEMENT INFORMATION RESOURCES

Books

AAHA Guide to Creating an Employee Handbook, American Animal Hospital Association, Denver, CO, 1992 (also available on computer disk)

Business of Veterinary Practice, The, John Sheridan and Owen McCafferty, Pergamon Press, Tarrytown, NY, 1993

How to Comply with Federal Employee Laws, Sheldon I. London, London Publishing Co., Washington, DC, 1991

Law and Ethics of the Veterinary Profession, James F. Wilson, DVM, JD, Priority Press Limited, Yardley, PA, 1988

Leadership & The One Minute Manager, Kenneth Blanchard, Patricia Zigarmi, and Drea Zigarmi, Berkeley Books, 1985

Management of Organizational Behavior, Paul Hersey and Kenneth Blanchard, Prentice Hall, Englewood Cliffs, NJ, 1982

Marketing of Professional Services, Francis G. Edwards, PennWell Publishing, Tulsa, OK, 1983

OSHA Compliance Guide for Veterinary Practices, American Aminal Hospital Association, Denver, CO, 1992

Power of Ethical Management, The, Kenneth Blanchard and Norman Vincent Peale, William Morrow and Co., New York, NY, 1988

Practice of Management, The, Peter F. Drucker, Harper and Row, New York, NY, 1954

Standard Abbreviations for Medical Records, American Animal Hospital Association, Denver, CO, 1992

Standard Chart of Accounts for Canadian Animal Hospitals, American Animal Hospital Association, Denver, CO, 1987

Successful Financial Management for the Veterinary Practice, Robert E. Froelich, DVM, MBA, American Animal Hospital Association, Denver, CO, 1987

Susan Lee's ABZ's of Economics, Susan Lee, Simon & Schuster, New York, NY, 1987

Type Talk, Otto Kroeger and Janet M. Thuesen, A Delta Book published by Dell Publishing, New York, NY, 1988

Veterinary Ethics, Jerrold Tannenbaum, MA, JD, William and Wilkins, Baltimore, MD, 1989

Veterinary Practice Management, Dennis McCurnin, DVM, J.B. Lippincott, Philadelphia, PA, 1988

Periodicals

DVM Newsmagazine, Edgell Communications Inc., Cleveland, OH

Harvard Business Review, James A. McGowan, Boston, MA

TRENDS Magazine, American Animal Hospital Association, Denver, CO

Veterinary Economics, Veterinary Medicine Publishing Company, Lenexa, KS

Veterinary Forum, Forum Publications Inc., Fairway, KS

Videotapes and Training Programs

OSHA Hazardous Material Training Program, American Animal Hospital Association, Denver, CO (training manual, required posters, and videotape)

SRI Support Services Perceiver Training, SRI Gallup, Lincoln, NE (a three-day training course on personality testing)

"The Telephone Doctor" Nancy J. Friedman, The Telephone Doctor, St. Louis, MO (videotape series on proper telephone use)

Veterinary Receptionist Videotape Series ("Telephone Techniques", First Impressions", "Special Situations"), American Aminal Hospital Association, Denver, CO

Veterinary Staff Training Videotapes ("Advanced Receptionist," "Dentistry and the Technician," "Radiology: Safety and Positioning"), American Animal Hospital Association, Denver, CO

Veterinary Management Development School, American Animal Hospital Association, Denver, CO (a four-day program held biannually in two levels)

Veterinary Management Institute, Purdue University, West Lafayette, IN and the American Animal Hospital Association, Denver, CO (an intensive, four-module residential study series offering over 72 hours of graduate-level instruction on contempory management issues)

Other Sources

American Animal Hospital Association, annual meeting, regional meetings, Veterinary Management Institute, Leading Edge Management Seminars, Practice Edge Management Reports. For information contact AAHA, Denver, CO, 800/252-2242 or 303/986-2800.

American Veterinary Medical Association, annual meeting and marketing seminars. For information contact AVMA, Schaumburg, IL, 800/248-2862.

Appendix B

PERSONNEL FORMS

JOB DESCRIPTION:

JOB DESCRIPTION FOR: ____________________

About the Job: ____________________

____

____

____

____

____

Job Requires: ____________________

____

____

____

____

____

Duties of Job: ____________________

____

____

____

____

____

____

Authority Boundaries: ____________________

____

____

____

____

____

Sample Job Description form

JOB DESCRIPTION FOR: Animal Hospital Receptionist

About the Job: The receptionist, answering the telephone to make appointments, greeting the clients when they arrive at the hospital, answering questions and concerns and collecting the fee as the client leaves the hospital will give the client the first and most lasting impression of the hospital. A satisfied client will, in most cases, indicate a satisfactory performance by the receptionist.

Job Requires: 1. A strong clear telephone voice and presence.

2. A liking of people and a willingness to work with them.

3. Adequate mathematic and spelling skills. (A test will be given)

4. Computers will be used. Data entry experience helpful but not required. Must be willing to learn.

5. Willingness to learn basic animal care facts and procedures.

6. Ability and willingness to be bonded.

7. Ability to work under stress.

8. Willingness to work 40 hours a week that includes 3 nights a week until 8 PM and every other Saturday from 8AM to 5PM.

Duties of Job: 1. Answer telephone, answer questions and concerns of clients and others and make appointments.

2. Receive clients and enter necessary data into computer.

3. Discharge patients after treatment or hospitalization, collect fees, and make necessary entries into computer and other financial records.

4. Safeguard funds and account for funds received while on duty.

5. File and account for medical records.

6. May be asked to handle an animal periodically.

7. Sell pet supplies offered by the hospital.

Authority Boundaries: Office Manager is responsible for hiring, training and evaluation. Salary increases, promotion and continued employment will be determined by the hospital owner on the recommendation of the Office Manager.

Sample Job Description for Receptionist

AAHA® AMERICAN ANIMAL HOSPITAL ASSOCIATION

APPLICATION FOR EMPLOYMENT

(PLEASE PRINT CLEARLY)

An Equal Opportunity Employer

We do not discriminate on the basis of race, religion, national origin, color, sex, age, veteran status, or disability. It is our intention that all qualified applicants be given equal opportunity and that selection decisions are based on job-related factors.

Personal

Social Security No. ____________ Date ____________

Name ______________________________
Last First Middle

Present address ______________________________ Telephone no. ____________
No. Street City State Zip

Position applied for ____________ Rate of pay expected $ ______ per week

Are you seeking ____ Full-time ____ Part-time Specify days and hours if part-time ____________

Were you previously employed by this organization? ____ If yes, when? ____________

List any friends or relatives working here, other than spouse ____________
Name(s)

If your application is considered favorably, on what date will you be available for work? ____________ 19 ____

Are there any other work experiences, skills, or qualifications that you feel would especially fit you for work here? Please add any additional comments you think are important for us to consider. ____________

If you are applying for a job with minimum age requirements, you may be required to submit proof of age.
For jobs with minimum age requirements:

Are you 18 years of age or older? . . . . . ☐ yes ☐ no

For driving jobs only: Do you have a valid driver's license? . . . . . ☐ yes ☐ no

Driver's license number ____________ Class of license ____________

Have you had your driver's license revoked or suspended in the last 3 years? . . . . . ☐ yes ☐ no

If hired, can you furnish proof you are eligible to work in the United States? . . . . . ☐ yes ☐ no

Have you ever been convicted of a felony? . . . . . ☐ yes ☐ no

A "yes" answer does not automatically disqualify you from employment since the nature of the offense, date, and the job for which you are applying will be considered.

If yes, please explain ____________

Have you previously applied here? . . . . . ☐ yes ☐ no

If yes, when? ____________

Have you worked for any firm under a different name? . . . . . ☐ yes ☐ no

If yes, give name ____________

Sample AAHA Employment Application form (page 1 of 4)

Personal References (not former employers or relatives)

Name and occupation	Address	Phone number

Membership in Professional or Civic Organizations (do not include racial, religious, or nationality groups)

Name or description of organization	Active participation		Offices held
	From	To	

Education Record—Nonveterinarians Only

Name of school	Degree awarded	Grade average	Honors
High School			
College or University			
Business, Trade, Correspondence, or Night School			
Other			

Do you type? ☐ Yes ☐ Manual machines ______ WPM ☐ No ☐ Electric machines ______ WPM	Shorthand ______ WPM	Office machines and computers you know how to operate

Education Record—Veterinarians Only

Name of school	Degree awarded	Grade average	Honors
High School			
College or University (Preveterinary)			
College (Veterinary Curriculum)			

Postgraduate training, including internships (include dates and degrees awarded, if any)
Are you board certified? ☐ Board eligible? ☐ Which specialty board?
List continuing education courses attended in the past 18 months
List the states in which you are licensed to practice along with license numbers:

Sample AAHA Employment Application form (page 2 of 4)

Work History (begin with the most recent, list all past employers, including any pertinent military experience)

Name of Company	Business address City State		Phone no.
Type of business	Immediate supervisor		Date employed From To
Exact job title	Earnings at hire	At termination	Reason for termination
Description of duties			

Name of Company	Business address City State		Phone no.
Type of business	Immediate supervisor		Date employed From To
Exact job title	Earnings at hire	At termination	Reason for termination
Description of duties			

Name of Company	Business address City State		Phone no.
Type of business	Immediate supervisor		Date employed From To
Exact job title	Earnings at hire	At termination	Reason for termination
Description of duties			

Name of Company	Business address City State		Phone no.
Type of business	Immediate supervisor		Date employed From To
Exact job title	Earnings at hire	At termination	Reason for termination
Description of duties			

Affidavit

Please Read Each Statement Carefully Before Signing

I certify that all information I have provided in this application is true and complete. I understand that any false information or omission may disqualify me from further consideration for employment and may result in my dismissal if discovered at a later date. I understand that the employer may request an investigative consumer report from a consumer reporting agency. This report may include information as to my character, reputation, personal characteristics and mode of living obtained from interviews with neighbors, friends, former employers, schools and others. I understand I have a right to make a written request within a reasonable time for the disclosure of the name and address of the consumer reporting agency so that I may obtain a complete disclosure of the nature and scope of the investigation. I authorize the investigation of any or all statements contained in this application and also authorize any person, school, current employer (except as previously noted), past employers and organizations named in this application to provide relevant information and opinions that may be useful in making a hiring decision. I release such persons and organizations from any legal liability in making such statements. I UNDERSTAND THAT THIS APPLICATION OR SUBSEQUENT EMPLOYMENT DOES NOT CREATE A CONTRACT OF EMPLOYMENT NOR GUARANTEE EMPLOYMENT FOR ANY DEFINITE PERIOD OF TIME. IF EMPLOYED, I UNDERSTAND THAT I HAVE BEEN HIRED AT THE WILL OF THE EMPLOYER AND MY EMPLOYMENT MAY BE TERMINATED AT ANY TIME, WITH OR WITHOUT CAUSE AND WITH OR WITHOUT NOTICE. I have read, understand, and by my signature consent to these statements.

Signature____________________ Date____________

This application for employment will remain active for a limited time. Ask the organization representative for details.

Sample AAHA Employment Application form (page 3 of 4)

FOR EMPLOYER'S USE ONLY

Reference Check

Date Called	Company Called	Person Contacted	Comments

Interview Results

AAHA®
AMERICAN ANIMAL HOSPITAL ASSOCIATION

Published as a membership service by the American Animal Hospital Association

"The objective of the AAHA is to improve the quality of medical care and service to pet animals and the pet-owning public by promoting the universal acceptance of high standards for all aspects of veterinary practice and to represent and speak out as the one voice for small animal veterinary medicine."

Sample AAHA Employment Application form (page 4 of 4)

FOR OFFICE USE ONLY	
Possible Work Locations	Possible Positions

APPLICATION FOR EMPLOYMENT

FOR OFFICE USE ONLY	
Work Location ____	Rate ____
Position ____	Date ____

(PLEASE PRINT PLAINLY)

PERSONAL

Date ____

Name ____ (Last, First, Middle) Social Security No. ____

Present address ____ (No., Street, City, State, Zip) Telephone No. ____

Are you legally eligible for employment in the U.S.A.? Yes___ No___ (If yes, verification will be required.)

Are you of the legal age to work? ____

Position(s) applied for ____

Were you previously employed by us?____ If yes, when? ____

If your application is considered favorably, on what date will you be available for work? ____ 19____

Are there any other experiences, skills, or qualifications which will be of special benefit in the job for which you are applying? (Applicant should not list any information that Federal and/or State law precludes obtaining in the pre-employment stage.) ____

RECORD OF EDUCATION

School	Name and Address of School	Course of Study	Check Last Year Completed	Did You Graduate?	List Diploma or Degree
Elementary		X	5 6 7 8	☐ Yes ☐ No	X
High			1 2 3 4	☐ Yes ☐ No	
College			1 2 3 4	☐ Yes ☐ No	
Other (Specify)			1 2 3 4	☐ Yes ☐ No	

(Turn to Next Page)

FORM 101

Sample Employment Application form (page 1 of 4)

List below present and past employment, beginning with your most recent

I

Name and Address of Company and Type of Business	From		To		Weekly Starting Salary	Weekly Last Salary	Reason for Leaving	Name of Supervisor
	Mo.	Yr.	Mo.	Yr.				
	Describe the work you did:							
Telephone								

II

Name and Address of Company and Type of Business	From		To		Weekly Starting Salary	Weekly Last Salary	Reason for Leaving	Name of Supervisor
	Mo.	Yr.	Mo.	Yr.				
	Describe the work you did:							
Telephone								

III

Name and Address of Company and Type of Business	From		To		Weekly Starting Salary	Weekly Last Salary	Reason for Leaving	Name of Supervisor
	Mo.	Yr.	Mo.	Yr.				
	Describe the work you did:							
Telephone								

IV

Name and Address of Company and Type of Business	From		To		Weekly Starting Salary	Weekly Last Salary	Reason for Leaving	Name of Supervisor
	Mo.	Yr.	Mo.	Yr.				
	Describe the work you did:							
Telephone								

I hereby give permission to contact the employers listed above concerning my prior work experience.

Signed ______________________________

If there is a particular employer(s), you do not wish us to contact, please indicate which one(s). ______________________________

____

PERSONAL REFERENCES (Not Former Employers or Relatives)

Name and Occupation	Address	Phone Number

—2—

Sample Employment Application form (page 2 of 4)

PLEASE READ AND SIGN BELOW

The facts set forth in my application for employment are true and complete. I understand that if employed, any false statement on this application may result in my dismissal. I further understand that this application is not and is not intended to be a contract of employment, nor does this application obligate the employer in any way if the employer decides to employ me. I understand and agree that my employment is at-will and can be terminated by either party with or without notice, at any time, for any reason or no reason. No one other than an officer of the Company has any authority to enter into any agreement for employment for any specified period of time or to make any agreement contrary to the foregoing and then only in a writing signed by an officer.

____
Signature of Applicant

To Applicant: READ THIS INTRODUCTION CAREFULLY BEFORE ANSWERING ANY QUESTIONS IN THIS BLOCKED-OFF AREA. The Civil Rights Act of 1964 prohibits discrimination in employment because of race, color, creed, religion, sex or national origin. Federal law also prohibits other types of discrimination such as age, citizenship, disability, veteran status, attainment of benefits, and participation in union activities. The laws of most states and many localities also prohibit some or all of the above types of discrimination as well as some additional types including, but not limited to, discrimination based upon ancestry, marital status, parental status, sexual orientation, or source of income. The Fair Credit Reporting Act imposes restrictions with respect to credit data.

DO NOT ANSWER ANY QUESTION CONTAINED IN THIS BLOCKED-OFF AREA UNLESS THE EMPLOYER HAS CHECKED THE BOX NEXT TO THE QUESTION, thereby indicating that for the position for which you are applying the requested information is needed for a legally permissible reason, including, without limitation, national security requirements, affirmative action, a bona fide occupational qualification or business necessity.

☐ Previous address ______________________________
No. Street City State Zip

☐ Are you over the age of eighteen? __________ If no, hire is subject to verification that you are of minimum legal age.

☐ Sex: M__________ F__________ ☐ Height:__________ ft.__________ in. ☐ Weight:__________ lbs.

☐ Are you a citizen of the U.S.A.? __________

☐ Were you in U.S. Armed Forces? Yes ______ No ______ If yes, what Branch? __________

☐ Did you receive any training in the U.S. Armed Forces that is relevant to the position applied for? (If yes, describe.) ______

____

☐ Are you a Vietnam veteran? __________

☐ Are you eligible to be bonded? __________

☐ Have you ever been convicted of a crime, excluding misdemeanors and summary offenses, in the past seven years which has not been annulled or expunged or sealed by a court? ______ If yes, describe in full __________

____

Conviction of a crime will not be an absolute bar to employment.

☐ You have been given a written job description listing the essential job functions of the position(s) for which you have applied. Please review the job description(s) and answer the following question. Are you able to perform each of the essential job functions listed for each position for which you have applied? ______ If no, list the function(s) you are unable to perform and explain why you are unable to perform them. __________

____

____

____

Employer may list other bona fide occupational questions on lines below:

☐ ______________________________

☐ ______________________________

☐ ______________________________

☐ ______________________________

—3—

Sample Employment Application form (page 3 of 4)

APPLICANT — Do not write on this page
FOR INTERVIEWER'S USE

INTERVIEWER	DATE	COMMENTS

FOR TEST ADMINISTRATOR'S USE

TESTS ADMINISTERED	DATE	RAW SCORE	RATING	COMMENTS AND INTERPRETATION

REFERENCE CHECK

*Position Number	RESULTS OF REFERENCE CHECK	*Position Number	RESULTS OF REFERENCE CHECK
I		IV	
II			
III			

***See Page 2**

This *"Application for Employment"* is prepared for general use throughout the United States. Our legal counsel has advised us that the material outside the blocked-off area complied with all Federal and State fair employment practice laws and with the Fair Credit Reporting Act. However, the various fair employment practice laws and related statutes and the interpretations of them change frequently, and neither V.W. Eimicke Associates, Inc. nor its counsel assume any responsibility for the inclusion in this *"Application for Employment"* of any questions that may violate local and/or State and/or Federal laws. Users should consult their counsel about any legal question they may have with respect to the use of this form.

—4—

Sample Employment Application form (page 4 of 4)

Application For Employment

NAME: ______ POSITION: ______ DATE: __/__/__

We consider applicants for all positions without regard to race, color, religion, creed, gender, national origin, age, disability, marital or veteran status, sexual orientation, or any other legally protected status.

(PLEASE PRINT)

Position(s) Applied For	Date of Application

How Did You Learn About Us?

☐ Advertisement ☐ Friend ☐ Walk-In
☐ Employment Agency ☐ Relative ☐ Other ______

Last Name	First Name	Middle Name

Address	*Number*	*Street*	*City*	*State*	*Zip Code*

Telephone Number(s)	Social Security Number

If you are under 18 years of age, can you provide required proof of your eligibility to work? ☐ Yes ☐ No

Have you ever filed an application with us before? ☐ Yes ☐ No

If Yes, give date ______

Have you ever been employed with us before? ☐ Yes ☐ No

If Yes, give date ______

Are you currently employed? ☐ Yes ☐ No

May we contact your present employer? ☐ Yes ☐ No

Are you prevented from lawfully becoming employed in this country because of Visa or Immigration Status? ☐ Yes ☐ No
Proof of citizenship or immigration status will be required upon employment.

On what date would you be available for work? ______

Are you available to work: ☐ Full Time ☐ Part Time ☐ Shift Work ☐ Temporary

Are you currently on "lay-off" status and subject to recall? ☐ Yes ☐ No

Can you travel if a job requires it? ☐ Yes ☐ No

Have you been convicted of a felony within the last 7 years? ☐ Yes ☐ No
Conviction will not necessarily disqualify an applicant from employment.

If Yes, please explain ______

WE ARE AN EQUAL OPPORTUNITY EMPLOYER

Sample Employment Application form (page 1 of 6)

Education

	Name and Address of School	Course of Study	Years Completed	Diploma Degree
Elementary School				
High School				
Undergraduate College				
Graduate Professional				
Other (Specify)				

Indicate any foreign languages you can speak, read and / or write			
	FLUENT	GOOD	FAIR
SPEAK			
READ			
WRITE			

Describe any specialized training, apprenticeship, skills and extra-curricular activities.

____

____

____

Describe any job-related training received in the United States military.

____

____

____

Sample Employment Application form (page 2 of 6)

Employment Experience

Start with your present or last job. Include any job-related military service assignments and volunteer activities. You may exclude organizations which indicate race, color, religion, gender, national origin, disabilities or other protected status.

			Dates Employed		Work Performed
1.	Employer		From	To	
	Address				
	Telephone Number(s)		Hourly Rate/Salary		
			Starting	Final	
	Job Title	Supervisor			
	Reason for Leaving				
			Dates Employed		Work Performed
2.	Employer		From	To	
	Address				
	Telephone Number(s)		Hourly Rate/Salary		
			Starting	Final	
	Job Title	Supervisor			
	Reason for Leaving				
			Dates Employed		Work Performed
3.	Employer		From	To	
	Address				
	Telephone Number(s)		Hourly Rate/Salary		
			Starting	Final	
	Job Title	Supervisor			
	Reason for Leaving				
			Dates Employed		Work Performed
4.	Employer		From	To	
	Address				
	Telephone Number(s)		Hourly Rate/Salary		
			Starting	Final	
	Job Title	Supervisor			
	Reason for Leaving				

If you need additional space, please continue on a separate sheet of paper.

List professional, trade, business or civic activities and offices held.
You may exclude membership which would reveal gender, race, religion, national origin, age, ancestry, disability or other protected status:

____

____

____

Sample Employment Application form (page 3 of 6)

Additional Information

Other Qualifications

Summarize special job-related skills and qualifications acquired from employment or other experience.

____

____

____

Specialized Skills   Check Skills/Equipment Operated

		Production/Mobile Machinery (list):	Other (list):
__CRT	__Fax		
__PC	__Lotus 1-2-3	________	________
__Calculator	__PBX System	________	________
__Typewriter	__Wordperfect	________	________
		________	________

State any additional information you feel may be helpful to us in considering your application.

____

____

____

Note to Applicants: DO NOT ANSWER THIS QUESTION UNLESS YOU HAVE BEEN INFORMED ABOUT THE REQUIREMENTS OF THE JOB FOR WHICH YOU ARE APPLYING.

Are you capable of performing in a reasonable manner, with or without a reasonable accommodation, the activities involved in the job or occupation for which you have applied? A description of the activities involved in such a job or occupation is attached. ____YES ____NO

References

1. ______________________________ (   ) ________
(Name) Phone #
____
(Address)

2. ______________________________ (   ) ________
(Name) Phone #
____
(Address)

3. ______________________________ (   ) ________
(Name) Phone #
____
(Address)

Sample Employment Application form (page 4 of 6)

FOR PERSONNEL DEPARTMENT USE ONLY

Position(s) Applied For Is Open: ☐ Yes ☐ No

Position(s) Considered For: ______________________

____

Date ____________

NOTES:

NAME: ____________ POSITION: ____________ DATE: ___ / ___ / ___

REV 3/93

Re-order Form #23960 (23962 imprinted) from Amsterdam Printing and Litho Corp., Amsterdam, N.Y. 12010

To Re-order Call 1-800-833-6231

Sample Employment Application form (page 5 of 6)

Applicant's Statement

I certify that answers given herein are true and complete to the best of my knowledge.

I authorize investigation of all statements contained in this application for employment as may be necessary in arriving at an employment decision.

This application for employment shall be considered active for a period of time not to exceed 45 days. Any applicant wishing to be considered for employment beyond this time period should inquire as to whether or not applications are being accepted at that time.

I hereby understand and acknowledge that, unless otherwise defined by applicable law, any employment relationship with this organization is of an *"at will"* nature, which means that the Employee may resign at any time and the Employer may discharge Employee at any time with or without cause. It is further understood that this *"at will"* employment relationship may not be changed by any written document or by conduct unless such change is specifically acknowledged in writing by an authorized executive of this organization.

In the event of employment, I understand that false or misleading information given in my application or interview(s) may result in discharge. I understand, also, that I am required to abide by all rules and regulations of the employer.

Signature of Applicant ____________________ Date ____________

FOR PERSONNEL DEPARTMENT USE ONLY

Arrange Interview ☐ Yes ☐ No

Remarks ______________________________

______________________________ INTERVIEWER ______ DATE

Employed ☐ Yes ☐ No Date of Employment ____________

Job Title ____________ Hourly Rate/ Salary ________ Department____________

By ______________________ NAME AND TITLE ______ DATE

NOTES ______________________________

This Application For Employment is sold for general use throughout the United States. Amsterdam Printing and Litho Corp. assumes no responsibility for the use of said form or any questions which, when asked by the employer of the job applicant, may violate State and/or Federal Law.

Sample Employment Application form (page 6 of 6)

1. Please circle the correctly spelled word in each group:

vetranarian	alleergy	hospitaleization
vetranary	allergy	hostilation
veterinarian	alergy	hospitalization
vetanarian	algre	hospitalizaeion
vetnarian	algery	hostalization

diarear	surgiery	consultation
diarrhea	surgry	consoltation
diarrhhea	sergery	consultition
diarhea	surgiry	
	surgery	

2. Please circle the letters found after the name of an animal doctor.

   a. PhD. b. M.D. c. D.V.M. d. D.D.S. e. V.M.D.

3. Make whatever corrections are necessary to make the following group of words an acceptable sentence.

   Because im hear today him and me can't go to the theater.

4. What does the word "euthanasia" mean?

5. The hospitalization fee for a dog is $18.00 per day. What would the charge be for an animal that has been in the hospital for 3 days? What would the charge be for 3 days plus surgery in the amount of $75.00?

   3 days________________________

   3 days + hospitalization________________________

Prospective Employee Test

SPELLING TEST

Correct the spelling of the following words, if appropriate

acomodate	__________	mispelled	__________
sincerely	__________	vetranarian	__________
inocent	__________	necessary	__________
temperary	__________	separate	__________
secratery	__________	surgry	__________
conscious	__________	antebiotic	__________
dictionry	__________	necessary	__________
alergy	__________	permanent	__________
grammer	__________	conclude	__________
misdemenr	__________	consoltation	__________

GRAMMAR TEST

Circle the word that would best complete the following sentences

1. Jan and ___ went to the library together

   a. me c. I
   b. she d. him

2. They are on ___ way to the meeting.

   a. there
   b. their
   c. they're

3. The building is entirely ___ tall

   a. to b. too c. two

4. Washington, DC is the nation's ___.

   a. capitol b. capital

5. Please order more office ___.

   a. stationary b. stationery

6. Mr. Clark is the ___ of the school.

   a. principal b. principle c. princeple

Prospective Employee Test

INTERVIEW CHECKLIST

Applicant Name	Date
Position Desired	Interviewer

Based on the requirements of the current position opening, check the appropriate box in each category, then make additional comments and recommendations below.

EXPERIENCE	JOB KNOWLEDGE	EDUCATION	MOTIVATION	EXPRESSION	APPEARANCE
☐ Background experience does not relate to current position opening.	☐ None as pertains to this position.	☐ No relevant educational background.	☐ None, apathetic, indifferent, disinterested.	☐ Uncommunicative confused thoughts, poor vocabulary.	☐ Indifferent to attire and grooming, sloppy, unkempt.
☐ Has little relative background experience, needs much training.	☐ Will need considerable training.	☐ Weak educational background.	☐ Doubtful interest in position.	☐ Poor speaker, hazy thoughts, ideas.	☐ Careless in attire, poor grooming.
☐ Has some relative background experience, needs some training.	☐ Basic, but will learn on the job.	☐ Some relevant educational background.	☐ Sincere desire to work.	☐ Speaks well, expresses ideas adequately.	☐ Functional attire, neatly groomed.
☐ Possesses adequate background experience, needs little training.	☐ Well versed in position, little training needed.	☐ Strong educational background.	☐ Strong interest in position, asks questions.	☐ Speaks, thinks clearly, with confidence.	☐ Well groomed.
☐ Background experience is exceptional match to job requirements.	☐ Extremely well versed, able to work without further training.	☐ Excellent educational background.	☐ Highly motivated, eager to work, asks many questions.	☐ Exceptional, speaks clearly, concisely with confidence, ideas well thought out.	☐ Immaculate attire and grooming.

OVERALL IMPRESSION ☐ Unsatisfactory ☐ Marginal ☐ Satisfactory ☐ Very Good ☐ Excellent

ADDITIONAL COMMENTS AND RECOMMENDATIONS

Should we interview further?	For what position?	Refer to: (Manager of position)	Department:

Interview Checklist form

TO: ____________________

FROM: ____________________

EMPLOYMENT INTERVIEW REPORT

NAME OF APPLICANT: ____________________ DATE OF THIS INTERVIEW: ____________________

ADDRESS ____________________ PHONE ____________________

CANDIDATE FOR ____________________ (Job Title)

INTERVIEWER: ____________________

THIS IS: 1st INTERVIEW ☐ 2nd INTERVIEW ☐ 3rd INTERVIEW ☐

PLEASE REPORT YOUR INTERVIEW IMPRESSIONS BY CHECKING THE ONE MOST APPROPRIATE BOX IN EACH AREA.

1. FRIENDLINESS (If relevant to the particular job.)				
Appears very distant and aloof. ☐	Approachable; fairly friendly. ☐	Warm; friendly; sociable. ☐	Very sociable and outgoing. ☐	Extremely friendly and sociable. ☐
2. POISE				
Ill at ease. ☐	Somewhat tense; is easily irritated. ☐	About as poised as the average applicant. ☐	Confident; appears to like crises more than average person. ☐	Extremely well composed; apparently thrives under pressure. ☐
3. PERSONALITY (An individual's personality traits as they relate to personal suitability for the job.)				
Unsatisfactory for this job. ☐	Questionable for this job. ☐	Satisfactory for this job. ☐	Very desirable for this job. ☐	Outstanding for this job. ☐
4. CONVERSATIONAL ABILITY (Only if an essential function of the particular job.)				
Talks very little; expression poor ☐	Attempts expression but does fair job at best. ☐	Average fluency and expression. ☐	Talks well and "to the point." ☐	Excellent expression; extremely fluent; forceful. ☐
5. APTITUDE				
Slow to "catch on." ☐	Rather slow; requires more than average explanation. ☐	Grasps ideas with average ability. ☐	Quick to understand; perceives very well. ☐	Exceptionally keen and quick-learning. ☐
6. INFORMATION ABOUT GENERAL WORK FIELD				
Poor knowledge of field. ☐	Fair knowledge of field. ☐	Is as informed as the average applicant. ☐	Fairly well informed; knows more than average applicant. ☐	Has excellent knowledge of the field. ☐
7. EXPERIENCE				
No relationship between applicant's background and job requirements. ☐	Fair relationship between applicant's background and job requirements. ☐	Average amount of meaningful background and experience. ☐	Background very good; considerable experience. ☐	Excellent background and experience. ☐
8. DRIVE				
Has poorly defined goals and appears to act without purpose. ☐	Appears to set goals too low and to put forth little effort to achieve these. ☐	Appears to have average goals; puts forth average effort to reach these. ☐	Appears to strive hard; has high desire to achieve. ☐	Appears to set high goals and to strive incessantly to achieve these. ☐
9. OVERALL				
Definitely unsatisfactory. ☐	Substandard. ☐	Average. ☐	Definitely above average. ☐	Outstanding. ☐

(PLEASE SEE REVERSE SIDE)

FORM 103

Interview Report form (page 1 of 2)

THIS APPLICANT SHOULD BE HIRED: YES ☐ NO ☐ IF NO, STATE REASON: ____________

IF NO, WOULD YOU RECOMMEND CONSIDERATION AT FUTURE DATE FOR THIS OR ANY OTHER POSITION?

YES ☐ NO ☐ REMARKS ____________

TYPE OF WORK FOR WHICH APPLICANT APPEARS BEST QUALIFIED: ____________

IF THIS APPLICANT HAS IDENTIFIED HIMSELF/HERSELF AS DISABLED AND HAS REQUESTED ACCOMMODATION, WHAT POSSIBLE ACCOMMODATIONS WERE DISCUSSED WITH THE APPLICANT?

ADDITIONAL COMMENTS: ____________

Interview Report form (page 2 of 2)

PRE-EMPLOYMENT REFERENCE CHECK

____________________19_____

____

____

____

Attention: ____________________________

The applicant named below has told us that he/she previously worked for your Company. We would appreciate your furnishing us with as much of the information requested below as possible. We assure you that any information you may give will be treated confidentially.

An early reply will be greatly appreciated.

Sincerely yours,

________________________ Title ________

Co. Name: ________________________

Co. Address: ________________________

APPLICANT'S NAME ________________________ SOCIAL SECURITY/ INSURANCE NUMBER* ____________

DATES IN YOUR EMPLOY: FROM____________ TO____________ SALARY: $________ PER________

POSITION HELD ____________________________________

Is the information listed above correct? YES________ NO________ If no, please supply the correct information below.

____

____

Why did applicant leave your Company?________________________

Would you re-employ? YES________ NO________ If no, why not?________________

____

____

Please rate applicant on the following characteristics:

	POOR	FAIR	AVERAGE	VERY GOOD	EXCELLENT
QUALITY OF WORK					
QUANTITY OF WORK					
SUITABILITY FOR POSITION					
ATTENDANCE					
DEPENDABILITY					
COOPERATIVENESS					
CREATIVENESS					

DATE________________ SIGNED________________________

____

TITLE

*In USA, use Social Security Number.
In Canada, use Social Insurance Number.

FORM 115

Reference Checking form

INDIVIDUAL PERFORMANCE EVALUATION

Employee: ______________________ **Period Covered:** __________

Evaluator: ______________________ **Date of Review:** __________

	Ready To Train Others	Competent	Needs Help
ATTITUDE			
* Treatment of Clients	____	____	____
* Cooperation with other staff	____	____	____
* Cooperation with doctors	____	____	____
* Willingness to share skills	____	____	____
* Ability to teach others	____	____	____
* Eagerness to learn	____	____	____
* Overall job attitude	____	____	____
EFFICIENCY & PROFESSIONAL SKILLS			
* Ability to communicate with staff	____	____	____
* Ability to communicate with clients	____	____	____
* Ability to anticipate veterinarian	____	____	____
* Work station maintenance	____	____	____
* Ability to stay productive	____	____	____
- even when it's a slow day	____	____	____
* Accuracy of reported information	____	____	____
* Healthcare charting proficiency	____	____	____
* Handling and restaining animals	____	____	____
* Knowledge of terminology	____	____	____
* Knowledge of safety factors	____	____	____
* Knowledge of medications	____	____	____
* Ability to learn	____	____	____
DEPENDABILITY			
* Punctuality	____	____	____
* Absenteeism	____	____	____
* Individual job tasks	____	____	____
* Pursuit of personal targets	____	____	____
* Support of practice goals	____	____	____

AREAS OF EMPLOYEE STRENGTHS: ______________________________

TARGET AREAS FOR PERSONAL ACTION: ______________________________

OTHER COMMENTS BY THE EMPLOYEE: ______________________________

Employee Receipt of Copy	Date	Evaluator's Signature	Date

Performance Evaluation form

EMPLOYEE EVALUATION FORM

NAME: ______________________________ DATE: ______________________

DEPARTMENT: ______________________________ JOB TITLE: ______________________

Purposes of this Employee Evaluation:

To take a personal inventory, to pin-point weaknesses and strengths and to outline and agree upon a practical improvement program. Periodically conducted, these Evaluations will provide a history of development and progress.

Instructions:

Listed below are a number of traits, abilities and characteristics that are important for success in business. Place an "X" mark on each rating scale, over the descriptive phrase which most nearly describes the person being rated. (If this form is being used for self-evaluation, you will be describing yourself.)

Carefully evaluate each of the qualities separately.

Two common mistakes in rating are: (1) A tendency to rate nearly everyone as "average" on every trait instead of being more critical in judgment. The rater should use the ends of the scale as well as the middle, and (2) The "Halo Effect," i.e., a tendency to rate the same individual "excellent" on every trait or "poor" on every trait based on the *overall* picture one has of the person being rated. However, each person has strong points and weak points and these should be indicated on the rating scale.

ACCURACY is the correctness of work duties performed.

Makes frequent errors.	Careless; makes recurrent errors.	Usually accurate; makes only average number of mistakes.	Requires little supervision; is exact and precise most of the time.	Requires absolute minimum of supervision; is almost always accurate.

APTITUDE is the ability to grasp instructions, to meet changing conditions and to solve novel or problem situations.

Slow to "catch on."	Requires more than average instructions and explanations.	Grasps instructions with average ability.	Usually quick to understand and learn.	Exceptionally keen and quick-learning.

CREATIVITY is talent for having new ideas, for finding new and better ways of doing things and for being imaginative.

Rarely has a new idea; is unimaginative.	Occasionally comes up with a new idea.	Has average imagination; has reasonable number of new ideas.	Frequently suggests new ways of doing things; is very imaginative.	Continually seeks new and better ways of doing things; is extremely imaginative.

Form 102

Performance Evaluation form (page 1 of 4)

***FRIENDLINESS** is the sociability and warmth which an individual imparts in his/her attitude toward customers, other employees, his/her supervisor and the persons he/she may supervise.

Very distant and aloof.	Approachable; friendly once known by others.	Warm; friendly; sociable.	Very sociable and out-going.	Extremely sociable; excellent at establishing good will.

PERSONALITY is an individual's personality traits as they relate to his/her personal suitability for the job.

Personality unsatisfactory for this job.	Personality questionable for this job.	Personality satisfactory for this job.	Very desirable personality for this job.	Outstanding personality for this job.

ATTENDANCE is faithfulness in coming to work daily and conforming to work hours.

Often absent without good excuse and/or frequently reports for work late.	Lax in attendance and/or reporting for work on time.	Usually present and on time.	Very prompt; regular in attendance.	Always regular and prompt; volunteers for overtime when needed.

HOUSEKEEPING is the orderliness and cleanliness in which an individual keeps his/her work area.

Disorderly or untidy.	Some tendency to be careless and untidy.	Ordinarily keeps work area fairly neat.	Quite conscientious about neatness and cleanliness.	Unusually neat, clean and orderly.

DEPENDABILITY is the ability to do required jobs well with a minimum of supervision.

Requires close supervision; is unreliable.	Sometimes requires prompting.	Usually takes care of necessary tasks and completes with reasonable promptness.	Requires little supervision; is reliable.	Requires absolute minimum of supervision.

DRIVE is the desire to attain goals, to achieve.

Has poorly defined goals and acts without purpose; puts forth practically no effort.	Sets goals too low; puts forth little effort to achieve.	Has average goals and usually puts forth effort to reach these.	Strives hard; has high desire to achieve.	Sets high goals and strives incessantly to reach these.

*If relevant to the particular job.

Performance Evaluation form (page 2 of 4)

JOB KNOWLEDGE is the information concerning work duties which an individual should know for a satisfactory job performance.

______	______	______	______	______
Poorly informed about work duties.	Lacks knowledge of some phases of work.	Moderately informed; can answer most common questions.	Understands all phases of work.	Has complete mastery of all phases of job.

QUANTITY OF WORK is the amount of work an individual does in a work day.

______	______	______	______	______
Does not meet minimum requirements.	Does just enough to get by.	Volume of work is satisfactory.	Very industrious; does more than is required.	Superior work production record.

PERFORMANCE UNDER PRESSURE is the ability to withstand pressure and to remain calm in crisis situations.

______	______	______	______	______
Cannot handle pressure; utterly incapable of performing job during crises.	Occasionally "blows up" under pressure; is easily irritated.	Has average tolerance for crises; usually remains calm.	Tolerates most pressure; very good tolerance for crises.	Thrives under pressure; really enjoys solving crises.

COURTESY is the polite attention an individual gives other people.

______	______	______	______	______
Blunt; discourteous; antagonistic.	Sometimes tactless.	Agreeable and pleasant.	Always very polite and willing to help.	Inspiring to others in being courteous and very pleasant.

OVERALL EVALUATION in comparison with other employees with the same length of service on this job:

______	______	______	______	______
Definitely unsatisfactory.	Substandard but making progress.	Doing an average job.	Definitely above average.	Outstanding.

Performance Evaluation form (page 3 of 4)

COMMENTS

Major weak points are—

1. ____________________
2. ____________________
3. ____________________

and these can be strengthened by doing the following:

Major strong points are—

1. ____________________
2. ____________________
3. ____________________

and these can be used more effectively by doing the following:

Rated by ____________________ *(Name)* ____________________ *(Title)*

(If not used as a self-evaluation form, the employee should sign below)

A copy of this Report has been given to me and has been discussed with me.

____________________ *(Employee's Signature)* ____________________ *(Date)*

Performance Evaluation form (page 4 of 4)

U.S. Department of Justice
Immigration and Naturalization Service

OMB No. 1115-0136
Employment Eligibility Verification

Please read instructions carefully before completing this form. The instructions must be available during completion of this form. ANTI-DISCRIMINATION NOTICE. It is illegal to discriminate against work eligible individuals. Employers CANNOT specify which document(s) they will accept from an employee. The refusal to hire an individual because of a future expiration date may also constitute illegal discrimination.

Section 1. Employee Information and Verification. To be completed and signed by employee at the time employment begins

Print Name: Last	First	Middle Initial	Maiden Name
Address *(Street Name and Number)*		Apt. #	Date of Birth *(month/day/year)*
City	State	Zip Code	Social Security #

I am aware that federal law provides for imprisonment and/or fines for false statements or use of false documents in connection with the completion of this form.

I attest, under penalty of perjury, that I am (check one of the following):
- ☐ A citizen or national of the United States
- ☐ A Lawful Permanent Resident (Alien # A________________
- ☐ An alien authorized to work until ____/____/____
  (Alien # or Admission #________________

Employee's Signature	Date *(month/day/year)*

Preparer and/or Translator Certification. *(To be completed and signed if Section 1 is prepared by a person other than the employee.) I attest, under penalty of perjury, that I have assisted in the completion of this form and that to the best of my knowledge the information is true and correct.*

Preparer's/Translator's Signature	Print Name
Address *(Street Name and Number, City, State, Zip Code)*	Date *(month/day/year)*

Section 2. Employer Review and Verification. To be completed and signed by employer. **Examine one document from List A OR examine one document from List B and one from List C** as listed on the reverse of this form and record the title, number and expiration date, if any, of the document(s)

	List A	OR	List B	AND	List C
Document title:	____________		____________		____________
Issuing authority:	____________		____________		____________
Document #:	____________		____________		____________
Expiration Date *(if any)*:	___/___/___		___/___/___		___/___/___
Document #:	____________				
Expiration Date *(if any)*:	___/___/___				

CERTIFICATION - I attest, under penalty of perjury, that I have examined the document(s) presented by the above-named employee, that the above-listed document(s) appear to be genuine and to relate to the employee named, that the employee began employment on *(month/day/year)* ____/____/____ **and that to the best of my knowledge the employee is eligible to work in the United States. (State employment agencies may omit the date the employee began employment).**

Signature of Employer or Authorized Representative	Print Name	Title
Business or Organization Name	Address *(Street Name and Number, City, State, Zip Code)*	Date *(month/day/year)*

Section 3. Updating and Reverification. To be completed and signed by employer

A. New Name *(if applicable)*	B. Date of rehire *(month/day/year) (if applicable)*

C. If employee's previous grant of work authorization has expired, provide the information below for the document that establishes current employment eligibility.

Document Title:________________ Document #:________________ Expiration Date (if any):___/___/___

I attest, under penalty of perjury, that to the best of my knowledge, this employee is eligible to work in the United States, and if the employee presented document(s), the document(s) I have examined appear to be genuine and to relate to the individual.

Signature of Employer or Authorized Representative	Date *(month/day/year)*

Form I-9 (Rev. 11-21-91) N

Employment Eligibility form (page 1 of 2)

U.S. Department of Justice
Immigration and Naturalization Service

OMB No. 1115-0136
Employment Eligibility Verification

INSTRUCTIONS

PLEASE READ ALL INSTRUCTIONS CAREFULLY BEFORE COMPLETING THIS FORM.

Anti-Discrimination Notice. It is illegal to discriminate against any individual (other than an alien not authorized to work in the U.S.) in hiring, discharging, or recruiting or referring for a fee because of that individual's national origin or citizenship status. It is illegal to discriminate against work eligible individuals. Employers **CANNOT** specify which document(s) they will accept from an employee. The refusal to hire an individual because of a future expiration date may also constitute illegal discrimination.

Section 1 - Employee. All employees, citizens and noncitizens, hired after November 6, 1986, must complete Section 1 of this form at the time of hire, which is the actual beginning of employment. **The employer is responsible for ensuring that Section 1 is timely and properly completed.**

Preparer/Translator Certification. The Preparer/Translator Certification must be completed if Section 1 is prepared by a person other than the employee. A preparer/translator may be used only when the employee is unable to complete Section 1 on his/her own. However, the employee must still sign Section 1 personally.

Section 2 - Employer. For the purpose of completing this form, the term "employer" includes those recruiters and referrers for a fee who are agricultural associations, agricultural employers, or farm labor contractors.

Employers must complete Section 2 by examining evidence of identity and employment eligibility within three (3) business days of the date employment begins. If employees are authorized to work, but are unable to present the required document(s) within three business days, they must present a receipt for the application of the document(s) within three business days and the actual document(s) within ninety (90) days. However, if employers hire individuals for a duration of less than three business days, Section 2 must be completed at the time employment begins. **Employers must record:** 1) document title; 2) issuing authority; 3) document number, 4) expiration date, if any; and 5) the date employment begins. Employers must sign and date the certification. Employees must present original documents. Employers may, but are not required to, photocopy the document(s) presented. These photocopies may only be used for the verification process and must be retained with the I-9. **However, employers are still responsible for completing the I-9.**

Section 3 - Updating and Reverification. Employers must complete Section 3 when updating and/or reverifying the I-9. Employers must reverify employment eligibility of their employees on or before the expiration date recorded in Section 1. Employers **CANNOT** specify which document(s) they will accept from an employee.

- If an employee's name has changed at the time this form is being updated/ reverified, complete Block A.
- If an employee is rehired within three (3) years of the date this form was originally completed and the employee is still eligible to be employed on the same basis as previously indicated on this form (updating), complete Block B and the signature block.
- If an employee is rehired within three (3) years of the date this form was originally completed and the employee's work authorization has expired **or** if a current employee's work authorization is about to expire (reverification), complete Block B and:
  - examine any document that reflects that the employee is authorized to work in the U.S. (see List A or C),
  - record the document title, document number and expiration date (if any) in Block C, and
  - complete the signature block.

Photocopying and Retaining Form I-9. A blank I-9 may be reproduced provided both sides are copied. The Instructions must be available to all employees completing this form. Employers must retain completed I-9s for three (3) years after the date of hire **or** one (1) year after the date employment ends, whichever is later.

For more detailed information, you may refer to the INS Handbook for Employers, (Form M-274). You may obtain the handbook at your local INS office.

Privacy Act Notice. The authority for collecting this information is the Immigration Reform and Control Act of 1986, Pub. L. 99-603 (8 U.S.C. 1324a).

This information is for employers to verify the eligibility of individuals for employment to preclude the unlawful hiring, or recruiting or referring for a fee, of aliens who are not authorized to work in the United States.

This information will be used by employers as a record of their basis for determining eligibility of an employee to work in the United States. The form will be kept by the employer and made available for inspection by officials of the U.S. Immigration and Naturalization Service, the Department of Labor, and the Office of Special Counsel for Immigration Related Unfair Employment Practices.

Submission of the information required in this form is voluntary. However, an individual may not begin employment unless this form is completed since employers are subject to civil or criminal penalties if they do not comply with the Immigration Reform and Control Act of 1986.

Reporting Burden. We try to create forms and instructions that are accurate, can be easily understood, and which impose the least possible burden on you to provide us with information. Often this is difficult because some immigration laws are very complex. Accordingly, the reporting burden for this collection of information is computed as follows: 1) learning about this form, 5 minutes; 2) completing the form, 5 minutes; and 3) assembling and filing (recordkeeping) the form, 5 minutes, for an average of 15 minutes per response. If you have comments regarding the accuracy of this burden estimate, or suggestions for making this form simpler, you can write to both the Immigration and Naturalization Service, 425 I Street, N.W., Room 5304, Washington, D. C. 20536; and the Office of Management and Budget, Paperwork Reduction Project, OMB No. 1115-0136, Washington, D.C. 20503.

Form I-9 (Rev. 11-21-91) N

EMPLOYERS MUST RETAIN COMPLETED I-9
PLEASE DO NOT MAIL COMPLETED I-9 TO INS

Employment Eligibility form (page 2 of 2)

Form W-4 (1994)

Want More Money In Your Paycheck? If you expect to be able to take the earned income credit for 1994, you can have part of it added to your take-home pay. For details, get Form W-5 from your employer.

Purpose. Complete Form W-4 so that your employer can withhold the correct amount of Federal income tax from your pay.

Exemption From Withholding. Read line 7 of the certificate below to see if you can claim exempt status. *If exempt, complete line 7; but do not complete lines 5 and 6.* No Federal income tax will be withheld from your pay. Your exemption is good for 1 year only. It expires February 15, 1995.

Note: *You cannot claim exemption from withholding if (1) your income exceeds $600 and includes unearned income (e.g., interest and dividends), and (2) another person can claim you as a dependent on their tax return.*

Basic Instructions. Employees who are not exempt should complete the Personal Allowances Worksheet. Additional worksheets are provided on page 2 for employees to adjust their withholding allowances based on itemized deductions, adjustments to income, or two-earner/two-job situations. Complete all worksheets that apply to your situation. The worksheets will help you figure the number of withholding allowances you are entitled to claim. However, you may claim fewer allowances than this.

Head of Household. Generally, you may claim head of household filing status on your tax return only if you are unmarried and pay more than 50% of the costs of keeping up a home for yourself and your dependent(s) or other qualifying individuals.

Nonwage Income. If you have a large amount of nonwage income, such as interest or dividends, you should consider making estimated tax payments using Form 1040-ES. Otherwise, you may find that you owe additional tax at the end of the year.

Two Earners/Two Jobs. If you have a working spouse or more than one job, figure the total number of allowances you are entitled to claim on all jobs using worksheets from only one Form W-4. This total should be divided among all jobs. Your withholding will usually be most accurate when all allowances are claimed on the W-4 filed for the highest paying job and zero allowances are claimed for the others.

Check Your Withholding. After your W-4 takes effect, you can use **Pub. 919,** Is My Withholding Correct for 1994?, to see how the dollar amount you are having withheld compares to your estimated total annual tax. We recommend you get Pub. 919 especially if you used the Two Earner/Two Job Worksheet and your earnings exceed $150,000 (Single) or $200,000 (Married). Call 1-800-829-3676 to order Pub. 919. Check your telephone directory for the IRS assistance number for further help.

Personal Allowances Worksheet

A Enter "1" for **yourself** if no one else can claim you as a dependent . . . . . **A** ______

B Enter "1" if:
- You are single and have only one job; or
- You are married, have only one job, and your spouse does not work; or
- Your wages from a second job or your spouse's wages (or the total of both) are $1,000 or less.

. . **B** ______

C Enter "1" for your **spouse.** But, you may choose to enter -0- if you are married and have either a working spouse or more than one job (this may help you avoid having too little tax withheld) . . . . . **C** ______

D Enter number of **dependents** (other than your spouse or yourself) whom you will claim on your tax return . . . . . **D** ______

E Enter "1" if you will file as **head of household** on your tax return (see conditions under **Head of Household** above) . **E** ______

F Enter "1" if you have at least $1,500 of **child or dependent care expenses** for which you plan to claim a credit . . **F** ______

G Add lines A through F and enter total here. **Note:** This amount may be different from the number of exemptions you claim on your return ▶ **G** ______

For accuracy, do all worksheets that apply.
- If you plan to **itemize or claim adjustments to income** and want to reduce your withholding, see the Deductions and Adjustments Worksheet on page 2.
- If you are **single** and have **more than one job** and your combined earnings from all jobs exceed $30,000 OR if you are **married** and have a **working spouse or more than one job,** and the combined earnings from all jobs exceed $50,000, see the Two-Earner/Two-Job Worksheet on page 2 if you want to avoid having too little tax withheld.
- If **neither** of the above situations applies, **stop here** and enter the number from line G on line 5 of Form W-4 below.

Cut here and give the certificate to your employer. Keep the top portion for your records.

Form **W-4**
Department of the Treasury
Internal Revenue Service

Employee's Withholding Allowance Certificate

▶ **For Privacy Act and Paperwork Reduction Act Notice, see reverse.**

OMB No. 1545-0010

1994

1 Type or print your first name and middle initial	Last name	2 Your social security number
Home address (number and street or rural route)	3 ☐ Single ☐ Married ☐ Married, but withhold at higher Single rate. **Note:** *If married, but legally separated, or spouse is a nonresident alien, check the Single box.*	
City or town, state, and ZIP code	4 If your last name differs from that on your social security card, check here and call 1-800-772-1213 for more information . . . . ▶ ☐	

5 Total number of allowances you are claiming (from line G above or from the worksheets on page 2 if they apply) . | 5 |

6 Additional amount, if any, you want withheld from each paycheck . . . . . | 6 | $

7 I claim exemption from withholding for 1994 and I certify that I meet **BOTH** of the following conditions for exemption:
- Last year I had a right to a refund of **ALL** Federal income tax withheld because I had **NO** tax liability; **AND**
- This year I expect a refund of **ALL** Federal income tax withheld because I expect to have **NO** tax liability.

If you meet both conditions, enter "EXEMPT" here . . . . . ▶ | 7 |

Under penalties of perjury, I certify that I am entitled to the number of withholding allowances claimed on this certificate or entitled to claim exempt status.

Employee's signature ▶ **Date** ▶ , 19

8 Employer's name and address (Employer: Complete 8 and 10 only if sending to the IRS)	9 Office code (optional)	10 Employer identification number

Cat. No. 10220Q

Form W-4 (page 1 of 2)

Form W-4 (1994) Page 2

Deductions and Adjustments Worksheet

Note: *Use this worksheet only if you plan to itemize deductions or claim adjustments to income on your 1994 tax return.*

1 Enter an estimate of your 1994 itemized deductions. These include: qualifying home mortgage interest, charitable contributions, state and local taxes (but not sales taxes), medical expenses in excess of 7.5% of your income, and miscellaneous deductions. (For 1994, you may have to reduce your itemized deductions if your income is over $111,800 ($55,900 if married filing separately). Get Pub. 919 for details.) . . . 1 $______

2 Enter: { $6,350 if married filing jointly or qualifying widow(er); $5,600 if head of household; $3,800 if single; $3,175 if married filing separately } . . . 2 $______

3 **Subtract** line 2 from line 1. If line 2 is greater than line 1, enter -0- . . . 3 $______

4 Enter an estimate of your 1994 adjustments to income. These include alimony paid and deductible IRA contributions 4 $______

5 **Add** lines 3 and 4 and enter the total . . . 5 $______

6 Enter an estimate of your 1994 nonwage income (such as dividends or interest) . . . 6 $______

7 **Subtract** line 6 from line 5. Enter the result, but not less than -0- . . . 7 $______

8 **Divide** the amount on line 7 by $2,500 and enter the result here. Drop any fraction . . . 8 ______

9 Enter the number from Personal Allowances Worksheet, line G, on page 1 . . . 9 ______

10 **Add** lines 8 and 9 and enter the total here. If you plan to use the Two-Earner/Two-Job Worksheet, also enter this total on line 1, below. Otherwise, **stop here** and enter this total on Form W-4, line 5, on page 1. . . . 10 ______

Two-Earner/Two-Job Worksheet

Note: *Use this worksheet only if the instructions for line G on page 1 direct you here.*

1 Enter the number from line G on page 1 (or from line 10 above if you used the Deductions and Adjustments Worksheet) 1 ______

2 Find the number in **Table 1** below that applies to the **LOWEST** paying job and enter it here . . . 2 ______

3 If line 1 is **GREATER THAN OR EQUAL TO** line 2, subtract line 2 from line 1. Enter the result here (if zero, enter -0-) and on Form W-4, line 5, on page 1. **DO NOT** use the rest of this worksheet . . . 3 ______

Note: *If line 1 is **LESS THAN** line 2, enter -0- on Form W-4, line 5, on page 1. Complete lines 4–9 to calculate the additional withholding amount necessary to avoid a year-end tax bill.*

4 Enter the number from line 2 of this worksheet . . . 4 ______

5 Enter the number from line 1 of this worksheet . . . 5 ______

6 **Subtract** line 5 from line 4 . . . 6 ______

7 Find the amount in **Table 2** below that applies to the **HIGHEST** paying job and enter it here . . . 7 $______

8 **Multiply** line 7 by line 6 and enter the result here. This is the additional annual withholding amount needed 8 $______

9 Divide line 8 by the number of pay periods remaining in 1994. (For example, divide by 26 if you are paid every other week and you complete this form in December 1993.) Enter the result here and on Form W-4, line 6, page 1. This is the additional amount to be withheld from each paycheck . . . 9 $

Table 1: Two-Earner/Two-Job Worksheet

Married Filing Jointly				All Others	
If wages from LOWEST paying job are—	Enter on line 2 above	If wages from LOWEST paying job are—	Enter on line 2 above	If wages from LOWEST paying job are—	Enter on line 2 above
0 - $3,000	0	39,001 - 50,000	9	0 - $4,000	0
3,001 - 6,000	1	50,001 - 55,000	10	4,001 - 10,000	1
6,001 - 11,000	2	55,001 - 60,000	11	10,001 - 14,000	2
11,001 - 16,000	3	60,001 - 70,000	12	14,001 - 19,000	3
16,001 - 21,000	4	70,001 - 80,000	13	19,001 - 23,000	4
21,001 - 27,000	5	80,001 - 90,000	14	23,001 - 45,000	5
27,001 - 31,000	6	90,001 and over	15	45,001 - 60,000	6
31,001 - 34,000	7			60,001 - 70,000	7
34,001 - 39,000	8			70,001 and over	8

Table 2: Two-Earner/Two-Job Worksheet

Married Filing Jointly		All Others	
If wages from HIGHEST paying job are—	Enter on line 7 above	If wages from HIGHEST paying job are—	Enter on line 7 above
0 - $ 50,000	$370	0 - $ 30,000	$370
50,001 - 100,000	690	30,001 - 60,000	690
100,001 - 130,000	760	60,001 - 110,000	760
130,001 - 220,000	880	110,001 - 220,000	880
220,001 and over	970	220,001 and over	970

Privacy Act and Paperwork Reduction Act Notice.—We ask for the information on this form to carry out the Internal Revenue laws of the United States. The Internal Revenue Code requires this information under sections 3402(f)(2)(A) and 6109 and their regulations. Failure to provide a completed form will result in your being treated as a single person who claims no withholding allowances. Routine uses of this information include giving it to the Department of Justice for civil and criminal litigation and to cities, states, and the District of Columbia for use in administering their tax laws.

The time needed to complete this form will vary depending on individual circumstances. The estimated average time is: **Recordkeeping** 46 min., **Learning about the law or the form** 10 min., **Preparing the form** 69 min. If you have comments concerning the accuracy of these time estimates or suggestions for making this form more simple, we would be happy to hear from you. You can write to both the **Internal Revenue Service,** Attention: Reports Clearance Officer, PC:FP, Washington, DC 20224; and the **Office of Management and Budget,** Paperwork Reduction Project (1545-0010), Washington, DC 20503. **DO NOT** send the tax form to either of these offices. Instead, give it to your employer.

Printed on recycled paper

☆ U.S. GOVERNMENT PRINTING OFFICE:1993-345-119

Form W-4 (page 2 of 2)

NEW-EMPLOYEE DATA CARD

Name ______________________________ Social Security No. __________
Last First Middle

IMPORTANT NOTICE The purpose of this form is to collect data for benefits and/or affirmative action reporting purposes and the information obtained will not be used for any other purpose including personnel or employment related decision-making.

The Civil Rights Act of 1964 prohibits discrimination in employment because of race, color, creed, religion, sex or national origin. Federal law also prohibits other types of discrimination such as age, citizenship, disability, veteran status, attainment of benefits, and participation in union activities. The laws of most states and many localities also prohibit some or all of the above types of discrimination as well as some additional types including, but not limited to, discrimination based upon ancestry, marital status, parental status, sexual orientation, or source of income. The Fair Credit Reporting Act imposes restrictions with respect to credit data.

IN CASE OF EMERGENCY NOTIFY

Name ______________________________ Telephone No. __________

Address ______________________________
No. Street City State Zip

ADDRESS

Present address ______________________________ Telephone No. __________
No. Street City State Zip

Previous address ______________________________ Telephone No. __________
No Street City State Zip

PERSONAL

Date of birth __________ Sex: M ____ F ____
Month Day Year

Marital Status: ______________________________ Date of marriage __________

Name of spouse ______________________________

Dependent children (Names and ages) ______________________________

______________________________ Number of dependents including yourself __________

RECORD OF EDUCATION

School	Name and Address of School	Course of Study	Check Last Year Completed	Did You Graduate?	List Diploma or Degree
Elementary			5 6 7 8	☐ Yes ☐ No	
High			1 2 3 4	☐ Yes ☐ No	
College			1 2 3 4	☐ Yes ☐ No	
Other (Specify)			1 2 3 4	☐ Yes ☐ No	

Name ____ Last ____ First ____ Middle ____

FORM 133

Printed in U S A

Employee Record form (page 1 of 2)

EMPLOYMENT HISTORY List below all past employment, beginning with most recent

Name and Address of Company and Type of Business	From		To		Weekly Starting Salary	Weekly Last Salary	Reason for Leaving	Name of Supervisor
	Mo.	Yr.	Mo.	Yr.				
	Describe the work you did:							
Telephone								

Name and Address of Company and Type of Business	From		To		Weekly Starting Salary	Weekly Last Salary	Reason for Leaving	Name of Supervisor
	Mo.	Yr.	Mo.	Yr.				
	Describe the work you did:							
Telephone								

Name and Address of Company and Type of Business	From		To		Weekly Starting Salary	Weekly Last Salary	Reason for Leaving	Name of Supervisor
	Mo.	Yr.	Mo.	Yr.				
	Describe the work you did:							
Telephone								

Name and Address of Company and Type of Business	From		To		Weekly Starting Salary	Weekly Last Salary	Reason for Leaving	Name of Supervisor
	Mo.	Yr.	Mo.	Yr.				
	Describe the work you did:							
Telephone								

Name and Address of Company and Type of Business	From		To		Weekly Starting Salary	Weekly Last Salary	Reason for Leaving	Name of Supervisor
	Mo.	Yr.	Mo.	Yr.				
	Describe the work you did:							
Telephone								

Name and Address of Company and Type of Business	From		To		Weekly Starting Salary	Weekly Last Salary	Reason for Leaving	Name of Supervisor
	Mo.	Yr.	Mo.	Yr.				
	Describe the work you did:							
Telephone								

The facts set forth above are true and complete to the best of my knowledge.

________________ Date   ________________________ Signature

Employee Record form (page 2 of 2)

1994 Attendance Controller™

Name ______________________________
Last First Middle

Employee/Payroll Number ______________ Dept. ______________

Hire Date __/__/__ Vacation days due ________ Sick days due ________

Telephone (______) ______________
Area Code

CODES

A - ACCIDENT
B - BIRTHDAY
C - PARTIAL HOURS WORKED
D - DEATH IN FAMILY
E - EXCUSED
F - ILLNESS-FAMILY
G - DISCIPLINE
H - HOLIDAY
I - ILLNESS-SELF
J - JURY DUTY
K - TRANSPORTATION
L - LEAVE OF ABSENCE
M - MILITARY
N - MEDICAL APPT.

P - PERSONAL
Q - LATE/EARLY QUIT
R - RECOGNITION
S - SUSPENSION
U - UNEXCUSED (AWOL)
V - VACATION
W - WEATHER
X - ACCIDENT OFF THE JOB
Z - LAYOFF
____ - ______________
____ - ______________
____ - ______________

LEGAL (FEDERAL) HOLIDAY

January

S	M	T	W	T	F	S	Days Used
						1	
2	3	4	5	6	7	8	
9	10	11	12	13	14	15	
16	17	18	19	20	21	22	
23 30	24 31	25	26	27	28	29	

January Totals (Days/Code) ______________

February

S	M	T	W	T	F	S	Days Used
		1	2	3	4	5	
6	7	8	9	10	11	12	
13	14	15	16	17	18	19	
20	21	22	23	24	25	26	
27	28						

February Totals (Days/Code) ______________

March

S	M	T	W	T	F	S	Days Used
		1	2	3	4	5	
6	7	8	9	10	11	12	
13	14	15	16	17	18	19	
20	21	22	23	24	25	26	
27	28	29	30	31			

March Totals (Days/Code) ______________

April

S	M	T	W	T	F	S	Days Used
					1	2	
3	4	5	6	7	8	9	
10	11	12	13	14	15	16	
17	18	19	20	21	22	23	
24	25	26	27	28	29	30	

April Totals (Days/Code) ______________

May

S	M	T	W	T	F	S	Days Used
1	2	3	4	5	6	7	
8	9	10	11	12	13	14	
15	16	17	18	19	20	21	
22	23	24	25	26	27	28	
29	30	31					

May Totals (Days/Code) ______________

June

S	M	T	W	T	F	S	Days Used
			1	2	3	4	
5	6	7	8	9	10	11	
12	13	14	15	16	17	18	
19	20	21	22	23	24	25	
26	27	28	29	30			

June Totals (Days/Code) ______________

July

S	M	T	W	T	F	S	Days Used
					1	2	
3	4	5	6	7	8	9	
10	11	12	13	14	15	16	
17	18	19	20	21	22	23	
24 31	25	26	27	28	29	30	

July Totals (Days/Code) ______________

August

S	M	T	W	T	F	S	Days Used
	1	2	3	4	5	6	
7	8	9	10	11	12	13	
14	15	16	17	18	19	20	
21	22	23	24	25	26	27	
28	29	30	31				

Aug. Totals (Days/Code) ______________

September

S	M	T	W	T	F	S	Days Used
				1	2	3	
4	5	6	7	8	9	10	
11	12	13	14	15	16	17	
18	19	20	21	22	23	24	
25	26	27	28	29	30		

Sep. Totals (Days/Code) ______________

October

S	M	T	W	T	F	S	Days Used
						1	
2	3	4	5	6	7	8	
9	10	11	12	13	14	15	
16	17	18	19	20	21	22	
23 30	24 31	25	26	27	28	29	

Oct. Totals (Days/Code) ______________

November

S	M	T	W	T	F	S	Days Used
		1	2	3	4	5	
6	7	8	9	10	11	12	
13	14	15	16	17	18	19	
20	21	22	23	24	25	26	
27	28	29	30				

Nov. Totals (Days/Code) ______________

December

S	M	T	W	T	F	S	Days Used
				1	2	3	
4	5	6	7	8	9	10	
11	12	13	14	15	16	17	
18	19	20	21	22	23	24	
25	26	27	28	29	30	31	

Dec. Totals (Days/Code) ______________

Employee Attendance form (page 1 of 2)

Summary of Employee Absence Information

Name ______________________ Position ______________________

Notes, Communications, Doctor Slips:

____
____
____
____
____
____
____
____
____
____

Quarterly Absence Totals:

Reason/ Code	First Qtr.	Second Qtr.	Third Qtr.	Fourth Qtr.	Year Total

Sick Time Allowed in 1994 ________
Carried over from 1993 ________

Vacation Time Earned for 1994 ________
Carried over from 1993 ________

	Sick Time			Vacation Time		
	Allowed	Taken	Available	Earned	Taken	Available
January						
February						
March						
April						
May						
June						
July						
August						
September						
October						
November						
December						

Warning Notices or Verbal Reprimands Given for Repeated Absences:

Date:			Comments:
/ /	☐ Verbal	☐ Warning Notice	______________________
/ /	☐ Verbal	☐ Warning Notice	______________________
/ /	☐ Verbal	☐ Warning Notice	______________________
/ /	☐ Verbal	☐ Warning Notice	______________________

FRIENDLY® FORMS

This Attendance Controller™ is to be retained in the employee's personnel file at the end of each year.

Employee Attendance form (page 2 of 2)

Company's Sexual Harassment Policy

Company is committed to providing a work environment for its employees free from sexual harassment. Intimidation or harassment based on sex is neither legal nor in keeping with the Company's philosophy of trust and mutual respect. Such action constitutes grounds for corrective discipline up to and including termination.

The Equal Employment Opportunity Commission's guidelines define sexual harassment as unwelcome sexual advances, requests for sexual favors or other verbal or physical conduct of a sexual nature when one or more of the following occur:

1. Submission or rejection of such conduct is made a term or condition of an individual's employment.
2. Submission or rejection of such conduct is used for the basis of an employment decision, such as promotion, demotion, termination, or pay.
3. Such condition interferes with an employee's work performance or creates a hostile, intimidating, or offensive work environment.

Examples of sexual harassment include, but are not limited to:

- making unwelcome comments about a person's clothing, body, or personal life;
- use of offensive nicknames or terms of endearment;
- telling offensive jokes or making inappropriate innuendoes;
- any suggestions that sexual activities would affect one's job, promotion, performance evaluation, or working conditions;
- unwanted overtures of a sexual nature; or
- other conduct that, even if not objectionable to some employees, creates a working environment that may be considered by others to be sexually hostile or offensive.

An employee who believes he/she is being harassed should take the following action:

1. If you are comfortable doing so, speak to the offender about his/her conduct. Explain that you do not like the conduct. The offensive conduct may have been thoughtless or based on a mistaken belief that it was welcome. In any event, respond immediately; do not ignore the problem.
2. If you are not satisfied with the result, notify your supervisor immediately.
3. If the offender is your supervisor, or if you are not comfortable speaking to your supervisor about the problem, speak to his/her superior, the Human Resources Department or the Plant Manager.
4. You also should immediately report any work-related harassment by a non-employee. Company will do its best to remedy the situation.

If a complaint is made, Company will conduct an investigation and take appropriate action. Confidentiality will be maintained to the extent possible without jeopardizing a full investigation. No employee will be disciplined or otherwise retaliated against for complaining about harassment.

Example Sexual Harassment policy

EMPLOYEE WARNING RECORD

Employee's Name ____________ Clock or Payroll No. ________ Dept. ________

Shift ____________ Time ________ a.m. p.m. Date of Warning ________

WARNING

Date of Violation ________
Time of Violation ________
Place Violation Occurred ________

NATURE OF VIOLATION
- ☐ Substandard Work
- ☐ Conduct
- ☐ Tardiness
- ☐ Uncooperative
- ☐ Carelessness
- ☐ Disobedience
- ☐ ________

COMPANY REMARKS

HAS EMPLOYEE BEEN WARNED PREVIOUSLY? ☐ YES ☐ NO	Form of Warning	WHEN WARNED and BY WHOM 1st Warning	2nd Warning	3rd Warning
	Oral			
	Written			

EMPLOYEE'S REMARKS RE: VIOLATION

The absence of any statement on the part of the EMPLOYEE indicates his/her agreement with the report as stated.

I have entered my version of the matter above.

Employee's Signature ____________ Date ________

ACTION TO BE TAKEN

Approved By ____________
Name Title Date

I have read this "warning" and understand it.

Employee's Signature ________ Date

Signature of person who prepared warning ________ Title ________ Date

DISTRIBUTION OF COPIES
- ☐ Employee
- ☐ Foreman or Supervisor
- ☐ Personnel Department
- ☐ Plant Manager

Supervisor's Signature ________ Date

Employee Warning form

EMPLOYEE WARNING REPORT

Employee's Name ______________ Date of Warning ________ Dept. ________ Shift ________

Clock or Payroll No. ________

Type of Violation

- ☐ Attendance
- ☐ Carelessness
- ☐ Disobedience
- ☐ Safety
- ☐ Tardiness
- ☐ Work Quality
- ☐ Other ________

WARNING

Violation: Date ________

Violation: Time ________ a.m. / p.m.

Place Violation Occurred ________

Company Statement

Employee Statement

Check Proper Box

☐ I concur with the Company's statement.

☐ I disagree with the Company's statement for the following reasons:

I have entered my statement of the above matter.

Employee's Signature ________ Date ________

Warning Decision

Approved By ________

Name — Title — Date

List All Previous Warnings Below

When Warned And By Whom

Previous Warning: **1st Warning**

Date ________

Verbal ________

Written ________

Previous Warning: **2nd Warning**

Date ________

Verbal ________

Written ________

Previous Warning: **3rd Warning**

Date ________

Verbal ________

Written ________

I have read this "warning decision" and understand it.

Employee's Signature ________ Date

Signature of person who prepared warning ________ Title ________ Date

Supervisor's Signature ________ Date

Copy Distribution

- ☐ Employee
- ☐ Personnel Dept.
- ☐ Supervisor
- ☐ Foreman
- ☐ Union Rep.

Employee Warning form

TERMINATION REPORT

EMPLOYEE NAME (Last)		(First)	(MI)
DEPARTMENT	TODAY'S DATE	TERMINATION EFFECTIVE DATE	LAST DAY WORKED
JOB TITLE	TERRITORY	CLOCK NO.	EMPLOYEE NO.

TYPE OF SEPARATION (Check One)

☐ Resignation (attach letter of resignation) ☐ Dismissal ☐ Retirement

☐ Mutual Agreement ☐ Layoff ☐ Other ________________

MAIL CHECK? ☐ Yes ☐ No

REASON FOR TERMINATION

☐ Absenteeism/Tardiness ☐ Job Change ☐ Insubordination ☐ Reduction In Force

☐ Health ☐ Incompetence ☐ Family ☐ Company Shut Down

☐ Other ____

____

Employee Evaluation (check appropriate boxes)

	Unsatisfactory	Fair	Satisfactory	Good	Excellent
Attendance					
Cooperation					
Initiative					
Job Knowledge					
Quality of Work					

Sample

Recommendation: ☐ Without Reservation ☐ With Some Reservation ☐ Would Not Recommend

Rehire? ☐ Yes ☐ No If No, Reason: ________________

ADDITIONAL COMMENTS

____

____

____

____

Signed ________________________ Date ________________

FOR OFFICE USE ONLY

Benefits Cancelled:

Life _____ Hospital _____ Other _________ Personnel Approval ___________ Date ________

Termination Report form

EXIT INTERVIEW

As an important part of the processing of your separation from employment with our company, we would appreciate a chance to review your honest and objective opinions regarding your work here. Feedback from our employees plays an important role in establishing and improving the conditions in our workplace and in evaluating our personnel.

I. PRELIMINARIES

Name	Hire Date
Position	Separation Date

The main reasons I am leaving employment here are:

A.

B.

C.

I am leaving to accept other employment ☐ Yes ☐ No

If yes, my new employer is: Starting Salary

My new position is:

What most influenced me to accept this new position was:

II. OVERALL SATISFACTION

Please check one:	Excellent	Good	Fair	Poor
Job Duties/Workload				
Salary				
Working Conditions				
Supervision				
Training/Orientation				
Company Policies				
Benefits				
Advancement Opportunities				
Company Image				

III. IMMEDIATE SUPERVISION & TRAINING

The job training and orientation I received by this company was:

CHECK ONE: ☐ Excellent ☐ Good ☐ Fair ☐ Poor

Comments:

My supervisor gave clear and understandable instructions:

CHECK ONE: ☐ Always ☐ Most of the time ☐ Sometimes ☐ Never

Comments:

I felt free to discuss my ideas and concerns with my immediate supervisor:

☐ Always ☐ Most of the time ☐ Sometimes ☐ Never

Exit Interview form (page 1 of 2)

I believe my immediate supervisor was fair and unbiased:

☐ Always ☐ Most of the time ☐ Sometimes ☐ Never

Comments:

IV. COMPENSATION AND WORKING CONDITIONS

I believe my salary here was:

☐ Excellent: Compares favorably with the marketplace.
☐ Average: Comparable with the marketplace.
☐ Poor: Not competitive with the marketplace.

I believe my fringe benefits were:

☐ Excellent: Compares favorably with the marketplace.
☐ Average: Comparable with the marketplace.
☐ Poor: Not competitive with the marketplace.

When I consider promotional opportunities that were available to me here, I think:

☐ There were many opportunities for advancement available to me.
☐ There were some, but not many opportunities for advancement available.
☐ There were very little, if any, opportunities for advancement available.

I feel that this company has been aware of the work I was doing and gave appropriate attention to my efforts and recognition for my achievements:

☐ Always ☐ Most of the time ☐ Sometimes ☐ Never

I found the workload to be fair:

☐ Always ☐ Most of the time ☐ Sometimes ☐ Never

Please describe what you liked best about working here:

Please list what you liked least about working here:

Would you recommend your friends to work here? ☐ Yes ☐ No

Thank you for your cooperation.

Employee

Date

Administrator

Date

Exit Interview form (page 2 of 2)

Americans with Disabilities Act
Information Sources

- **Americans with Disabilities Act: How will it affect your practice?**
  Journal of the American Veterinary Medical Association, Vol 200 No. 1, January 1, 1992 and Vol 200 No. 2, January 15, 1992

- **What Business Must Know About the Americans with Disabilities Act**
  A booklet available from the U.S. Chamber of Commerce, 1615 H. St. NW, Washington, DC, 20062, 800/638-6582.

- **Compliance Guide to the Americans with Disabilities Act Small Business Legislative Council**
  1156 15th St. NW, Washington, DC 20005

- **ADA: —Your Employment Rights as an Individual**
  ADA: —Your Responsibilities as an Employer
  Questions and Answers on the ADA
  All available from the Equal Employment Opportunities Commission, 1801 L St. NW, Washington, DC 20507, 800/669-EEOC (Title I).

- **ADA Handbook (Title I)**
  U.S. Department of Justice - 800/514-0301

- **ADA Technical Assistance Manual (Title I)** - cost is $25.00
  Superintendent of Documents, P.O. Box 37195, Pittsburgh, PA 15250

- **U.S. Architectural and Transportation Barriers Compliance Board**
  1111 18th St. NW, Suite 501, Washington, DC 20036, 800/USA-ABLE.
  Several booklets and services are available on Title III.

- **Presidents Committee on Employment of People with Disabilities** - 800/526-7234

Americans with Disabilities Act Information Sources

Appendix C

FRONT OFFICE FORMS

FRONT OFFICE SYSTEMS/AAHA 2.

Telephone - Policy & Procedures

			TYPE OF CALL					
			PATIENT					
		DISPOSITION OF CALL	EMERGENCY	NON-EMERGENCY	NON-MEDICAL	OTHER DOCTORS	BUSINESS CALLS	PERSONAL CALLS
DOCTOR IS IN THE OFFICE	1	Immediately, my aide will interrupt me and I will handle the call						
	2	Immediately, my aide will interrupt me but she will handle the call						
	3	Immediately, my aide will interrupt me but I will instruct her that I will handle the call when I finish what I'm doing						
	4	I will speak to callers only during certain hours or time periods						
	5	My aide will keep a list of incoming calls and I will return the calls in clusters whenever I get time free						
	6	My aide keeps a list and I will return calls at a scheduled time. My aide will instruct callers when to expect call						
	7	My aide will return the calls after she has spoken with me when I'm not busy						
	8	My aide will handle the calls without any direction from me						
DOCTOR OUT	9	My aide will contact me immediately and I will determine proper disposition						
	10	My aide will accumulate calls and I will dispose of the calls following my "in office" routine						

Sample Telephone Policy & Procedures form

FRONT OFFICE SYSTEMS/AAHA 8.

Telephone - Analysis Sheet

	Appointments	Continuing Medical Problem Questions	Other Hospitals or Other Doctors	Personal	Other
8 - 9					
9 - 10					
10 - 11					
11 - 12					
12 - 1					
1 - 2					
2 - 3					
3 - 4					
4 - 5					
5 - 6					
TOTAL					

Sample Telephone Analysis form

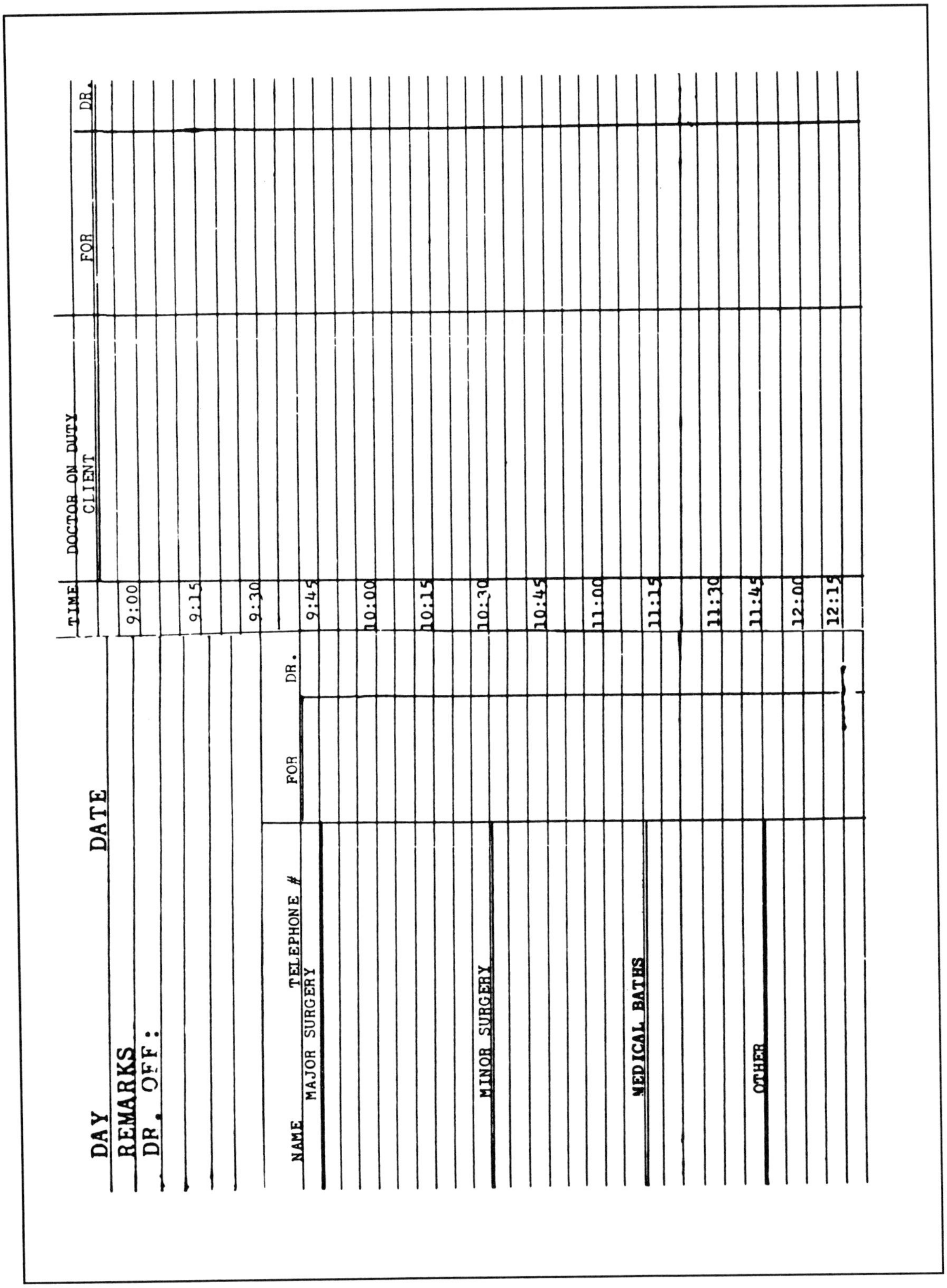
DAY DATE
REMARKS
DR. OFF:

NAME	TELEPHONE #	FOR	DR.
MAJOR SURGERY			
MINOR SURGERY			
MEDICAL BATHS			
OTHER			

TIME	DOCTOR ON DUTY CLIENT	FOR	DR.
9:00			
9:15			
9:30			
9:45			
10:00			
10:15			
10:30			
10:45			
11:00			
11:15			
11:30			
11:45			
12:00			
12:15			

Sample Appointment Schedule form (page 1 of 2)

DOCTORS ON DUTY

	CLIENT	FOR	DR.
12:30			
12:45			
1:00			
1:15			
1:30			
1:45			
2:00			
2:15			
2:30			
2:45			
3:00			
3:15			
3:30			
3:45			

DOCTOR ON DUTY

TIME	CLIENT	FOR	DR.
4:00			
4:15			
4:30			
4:45			
5:00			
5:15			
6:00			
6:15			
6:30			
6:45			
7:00			
7:15			
7:30			
7:45			
8:00			

Sample Appointment Schedule form (page 2 of 2)

AAHA®
AMERICAN ANIMAL HOSPITAL ASSOCIATION

Patient/Client Information

Thank you for giving us this opportunity to care for your pet. Please help us meet your needs better by taking a moment to complete both sides of this information sheet.

Date ____________________

Owner's Name ____________________ Spouse/Other____________________

Children (first name & ages) ____________________

Address ____________________ State/Prov. __________ Zip/PC__________

Home Telephone____________________ Work Telephone ____________________

Employer's Name & Address ____________________

Spouse's/Other's Employer & Address ____________________

At what time ________ and at what phone number ____________ is it best to call about your pet?

In case of EMERGENCY, please call ____________________ at phone number ____________

We will gladly prepare a written estimate if you desire. Please ask the receptionist or doctor.
PROFESSIONAL FEES ARE DUE AT THE TIME SERVICES ARE RENDERED.
If you pay by check or credit card, please complete the following (if state law allows):

Credit Card ____________ Acct. number ____________________ Expires ________

Personal Check __________ Driver's License: State/Prov. __________ Number________

Signature____________________

How did you first hear of our hospital? ❒ AAHA referral

❒ Individual: someone we may thank? ____________________ ❒ Hospital sign

❒ Yellow Pages for location ❒ Yellow Pages for service(s) ❒ Other ____________

We consider our pet(s) ❒ Part of the family ❒ just as pets

❒ Please add my name to your mailing list.

TO PREVENT THE SPREAD OF INFECTIOUS DISEASES AND PARASITES, HOSPITALIZED AND BOARDED ANIMALS MUST BE CURRENT ON ALL VACCINES AND FREE OF INTERNAL AND EXTERNAL PARASITES. I authorize the doctor to provide vaccines and parasite control as needed for my pet.

X ____

COMMENTS:____

____

____

Sample Patient/Client Information form (page 1 of 2)

ANIMAL MEDICAL HISTORY (please complete all information for each pet)

	PET #1	PET #2	PET #3
Name			
Species (cat, dog, other)			
Breed			
Description (color)			
Age (years)			
Date of Birth			
Sex			
Length of Time Owned			
Altered or Spayed			
Vitamins (type)			
Diet (kind of pet food)			
Type of Grooming Products			
Hours Spent Outside Each Day			
VACCINATIONS			
DHLP (distemper-dog)			
Parvovirus (dog)			
FVRCP (infectious diseases-cat)			
Rabies (dog/cat)			
Feline Leukemia Test			
Other Vaccines			
Heartworm Test			
Heartworm Prevention			
Fecal Exam (worms-dog/cat)			
Dentistry			
Prior Illness			
Prior Surgery			

PET ORIGIN: ❒ Humane Society ❒ Pet Shop ❒ Kennel ❒ Advertisement
❒ Friend ❒ Stray ❒ Individual (nonbreeder)

American Animal Hospital Association

Sample Patient/Client Information form (page 2 of 2)

American Animal Hospital Association

1 2 3 4 5 6 7 8 9 10 11 12 13 **Patient Data**

Owner's Name ______________________ Pet's Name ______________________

Address ______________________ City ______________________

State/Prov ______________________ Zip/PC ______________________

Phone: (H) ______________ (B) ______________ Breed ______________

Color ______________ Born ______________ Sex ______________

Idiosyncrasis ____

Health Maintenance	Date ☛											
Rabies												
Distemper/Respir Multivalent Vac												
FIP/Corona Vac												
FeLV/Parvo Vac												
FTLV/Bordetella Vac												
Annual Physical												
Heartworm Test/FeLV Test												
Fecal Exam												
Weight												
Dental Hygiene												
Diet												
Surgery Date												
X-ray Date												

ALERT DATA:

Date	#	Problem List	Resolved	Date	Medications

Sample Patient Data form

AAHA AMERICAN ANIMAL HOSPITAL ASSOCIATION

CLIENT SURVEY

Thank you for giving us the opportunity to serve you. Please help us better meet your needs by taking a moment to complete this questionnaire, and returning it to the receptionist or mailing it to our office.

	Yes	No
1. Was your call answered promptly?		
2. Was our telephone response courteous and helpful?		
3. Was our waiting room comfortable & clean?		
4. Did your wait before seeing the doctor seem brief?		
If not, how can we improve?		
5. Was the veterinary technician helpful and careful with your pet?		
6. Was the doctor courteous and genuinely concerned with your pet's health?		
7. Did the veterinarian explain your pet's problem clearly and completely?		
8. Do you feel your pet received quality professional health care?		
9. Did you find the facilty clean?		
10. If your pet was hospitalized, did the stay seem reasonable for the illness?		
11. After a hospital stay, was your pet returned to you clean?		
12. Was our payment policy clearly communicated to you?		
13. Was the billing presented in adequate detail?		
14. Would you recommend our veterinary practice to your friends?		
15. If your pet was groomed here, were you pleased?		

COMMENTS THAT YOU FEEL WOULD HELP OUR PRACTICE: ______________________________

____

____

____

____

____

Date service provided ________ Your name (optional) ______________ Pet's name ________________

#217 1/90

Sample Client Survey form

PRACTICE DEVELOPMENT TECHNIQUES/AAHA 7.

Client Satisfaction Survey

		Excellent	Good	Fair	Poor
1.	My overall satisfaction with this office visit is:				
2.	Our promptness in answering the telephone is:				
3.	The length of time spent "on hold" is:				
4.	The availability of our staff in an emergency is:				
5.	The realiability and courtesy of our answering service is:				
6.	The availability of convenient appointments is:				
7.	The time spent waiting to see our doctors is:				
8.	The quality of our business office staff is:				
9.	The quality of our technical staff is:				
10.	How do you feel about our veterinary care?				
11.	The cleanliness of our facility is:				

12. COMMENTS: ______________________________

____

____

____

____

Sample Client Survey form

Appendix D

COMPUTER DATA AND CREDIT INFORMATION FORMS

APPT.: ______________ ARRIVAL: ______________ CANINE FELINE

NO.: ______________ OWNER: ______________ PET: ______________ CASE. NO.

1 CASH
CHECK
2 M.CARD
VISA
3 DISCOVEF
CHG.

95

A. PROBLEM CODES: (C/R = TREATED, U = NOT TREATED, R = NOT WANTED)

_______ _______ _______ _______ _______ _______ _______

$ ______________

OFFICE VISITS

1. 1 PET
2. 2 PETS
3. 3 PETS
4. LITTER
5. DONNA L
6. RECHECK

7. FOLLOWUP
8. N/C
9. EMERGENCY
12. SPCA
13. SKIN REC
14. 4+ PETS

1D 7D 1S 1SL OVN OVG

1F 7F 1M WT SCRIPT #______________

VACCINES

15. DIST-C __
16. DIST-F __
17. FELV __
18. C-RAB __
19. F-RAB __

400.FROMMD __
401.NARAMU __
403.IMRABI __

LABORATORY

21. FECAL
60. VAG.SM.
23. URINE
24. U.SED
25. HW
11. FILTER
22. TAIL/DEW

28. CBC
29. STAIN
30. GLU
31. FELV/FV
26. HW TB
33. CYSTO
37. TAILS

34. C/S
27. P.M.
36. CULT/S
38. SCRAPE
39. HCT
341.DIL.INSULIN
40. DEWCLAWS

PROCEDURES

41. NAILS
42. TORN N
43. GLANDS
54. GL.N/C
44. EARS
53. EARS N/C
72. CLIP TREAT
46. EUTH
S M L XL

47. NAILS N/C
48. TORN DEWCL.
49. REMOVE DRAIN
50. TARTAR
51. TARTAR N/C
405.NOVALMITE TREAT
342.FLEA TREAT.
52. CREM
S M L XL

INJECTIONS
84. -ACEI
61. -ACTH
62. -AMBIPEN
64. -AMOXI
409. -BAYTRI
68. -CENTI
69. -DEPO
71. -DRONI
354. -IVOMEC
74. -LSXI
76. -OXY
77. -PENAQ
78. -PREDI
82. -VETI

ANTIBIOTIC
91. -AMOXD
92. -AMOX50
93. -AMOX100
110. -AMOX150
94. -AMOX200
369. -AMOX400
98. -AMP250
99. -AMP500
376. -BAYTRI20
377. -BAYTRI60
88. -CEFA 100
89. -CEFA 200

MISC. DRUGS
318. -ACE10
319. -ACE25
245. -DES
332. -LAXATONE
241. -NUTRI
408. -PHENL25
331. -URECH
440. -TORB5

PILLS
111. -CLAVAD
103. -CLAVA62
104. -CLAVA250
97. -CHPC500
240. -METRON
322. -OXA250
323. -OXA500
106. -PRIMOR120
107. -PRIMOR600
108. -SULFA500
437. -ANTI25
421. -ANTID

INTESTINAL
170. -ALBON
174. -CENT
175. -FORBID

FLEAS
144 -BASUS
368 -FLEA MOUS
430 -OVITROL16
428 -OVITROL32
125P-PRO10
126P-PRO20
127P-PRO40
128P-PRO80
379P-PRO160
129 -PROBAN
413 -PROBAN F
330 -PROBANL
138 -SIPH 6
139 -SIPH 2
384 -SIPHPAREA
442. -FLEA COMB

OINTMENTS
356 -CLEARX
183 -GOOD
184 -LIQUI
402 -NOLVA
429 -OXYDEX
187 -PANAC
189 -PANA15
190 -SYNO
399 -TOPAGEN
192 -TRES15
441 -OTOMAX

EYE OINTMENT
179 -ATROO
181 -CHLOROO
186 -NEOPRED

HEART
200. -THEO100
203. -LANOXIN
204. -COUGH
205. -LASIX12
206. -LASIX50

VITAMINS
214. -PTAB300
210. -FAVOR
216.-PTAB650
213.-PETTABS
388.-PETTINIC

STEROIDS
124 -CHLOR
116 -OVA5 R
118 -PSOLONE R
119 -PSONE20 R
123 -PSONE5 R
122 -PSOLONEF
353 -TRIAM 1.5
121 -VET 0.5

WORM MED
220 -DRONC
221 -DRONF
417 -PANA10
418 -PANA20
419 -PANA40
226 -VERCOM
432 -PYRA10
434 -PYRA50

SKIN
150 -ALLERGROOM
373. -RELIEF
160 -BITTER
344 -CHOLSHAM
433 -DERMSHAM
340 -DERMAHC 2
151 -EPISOOTH
431 -FLEASHAM
412 -ALLERSEB
224 -T-LUX
435 -DERM60
436 -DERMES60

HEARTWORM
309__ -GARD 25
310__ -GARD 50
311__ -GARD 100
385__ -GARDP25
386__ -GARDP50
387__ -GARDP100

EYE DROPS
324. -ATROD
325. -CHLOROD
326. -DEXAD
327. -GENTAD
193. -TEARS

438. -SYR3
439. -VACNEED

DRUG		AMOUNT	DOSE	COMMENT
______	______________	________	____ / ____	______________________
______	______________	________	____ / ____	______________________
______	______________	________	____ / ____	______________________
______	______________	________	____ / ____	______________________
______	______________	________	____ / ____	______________________
______	______________	________	____ / ____	______________________
______	______________	________	____ / ____	______________________

WHT: ______________ (______________)

I. RETURN VISIT
DATE TIME REASON
____/____/____ ______ ______

J. CALL BACK
DATE REASON
____/____/____ ______

K. RECHECK CARD
DATE REASON
____/____/____ ______

L. MESSAGES:

____ ____ ____ ____ ____ ____ ____ ____

51. ______________________________________

M. CERTIFICATES
47. HEALTH
48. NEUTER
50. RABIES

N. NOTATIONS: ______________________________________

____

____

____

Sample Computer Data form (page 1 of 2)

NO.:________________ OWNER:________________________________ DATE:______________

PET:________________ CANINE FELINE

1ST DISTEMPER

2ND DISTEMPER

3RD DISTEMPER

BOOSTER DIST.

FELEUK

RABIES

HW CK

H. CERT.

NAILS

SKIN

EARS

GLANDS

FECAL

COMPLAINT

____

____

____

____

____

____

____

____

____

____

____

TEMP: N______

PULSE:N______

RESP: N______

WEIGHT: ______

OUT-PATIENT

IN-PATIENT

REFERRED:

____

SYSTEM	NORMAL	AREA	SIGNS				COMMENTS
A. GENERAL	(YES)	1. WEIGHT CHANGE:	A. INCREASE	B. DECREASE			
		2. BODY CONDITION:	A. THIN	B. OVERWEIGHT	C. UNTHRIFTY		
	NO	3. ATTITUDE:	A. HYPERACTIVE	B. DEPRESSED			
B. INTEGU-MENTARY		1. SKIN:	A. >PIGMENT	B. EXCEMA	C. PISTULES	D. DRY	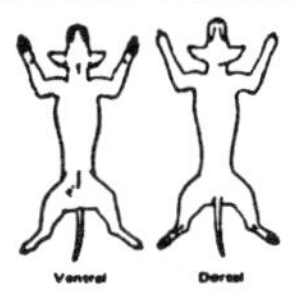
	(YES)		E. VESTICLES	F. EXCORIATION	G. DANDRUFF	H. TUMOR	
			I. SEBORRHEA	J. LACERATION	K. GRANULOMA	L. CYST	
			M. GRANULOMA	N. ABCESS	O. HEMATOMA		
			1. LOCAL	2. GENERAL	3. SEASONAL		
		2. HAIRCOAT:	A. ALOPECIA	B. >SHEDDING	C. DULL		
	NO		D. RETAINED	E. MATTED			
		3. PARASITES:	A. FLEAS	B. MITES	C. TICKS	D. LICE	
		4. ANAL GLANDS:	A. INFECTED	B. IMPACTED	C. ABESSED	D. TUMOR	
		5. FEET:	A. LACERATION	B. CYSTS	C. INFECTED		
		6. NAILS:	A. OVERGROWN	B. TORN	C. INFECTED		
		7. DEHYDRATION:	A. MODERATE	B. SEVERE			
C. MUSCULO-SKELETAL	(YES)	1. POSTURE:	A. VARUS	B. VELGUS	C. HYPEREXT.		
			D. HYPERFLEX	E. MUSCLE DYSTRO			
		2. GAIT:	A. LIMP	B. NON-WT.BEAR			
	NO		1. RF	2. LF	3. RR	4. LR	
		3. PAIN:	A. NECK	B. BACK	C. JOINT	D. MUSCLE	
D. DIGESTIVE		1. SIGNS:	A. VOMITING	B. DIARRHEA	C. CONSTIPAT.		
		2. APPETITE:	A. INCREASED	B. DECREASED	C. NONE		
	(YES)	3. LIPS	A. INFLAMMED	B. INFECTED	C. ULCERATED	D. EDEMA	
		4. MOUTH:	A. INFLAMMED	B. INFECTED	C. ULCERATED	D. TUMOR	
		5. TONGUE:	A. INFLAMMED	B. INFECTED	C. ULCERATED	D. TUMOR	
			E. SWOLLEN	F. LACERATED			
		6. GUMS:	A. INFLAMMED	B. INFECTED	C. PALE	D. PETECCH	
		7. TEETH:	A. INFECTED	B. TARTAR	C. DECIDUOUS		
	NO	8. TONSILS & PHARN:	A. INFAMMED	B. INFECTED	C. ENLARGED	D TUMOR	
		9. SALIVARY GLANDS:	A. ENLARGED	B. PAINFUL	C. INFECTED	D. TUMOR	
		10. AUSCULTATION:	A.________				
		11. PERCUSSION:	A.________				
E. RESPIR-ATORY		1. SIGNS:	A. SNEEZING	B. GAGGING	C. DYSPNEA		
			D. NASAL DISCHARGE		E. NASAL SWELL		
	(YES)	2. LARYNX:	A. INFLAMMED	B. INFECTED	C. SWOLLEN		
		3. COUGH:	A. EXCITEMENT	B. NOCTURNAL	C. SOFT	D. DRY	
			E. PRODUCTIVE	F. CONTINUOUS	G. PERIODIC	H. INDUCT	
	NO	4. AUSCULATATION:	A.________				
		5. PERCUSSION:	A.________				
F. EYES		1. SIGNS:	A. PAINFUL	B. SQUINTING	C. CLOSED	D. PROPTES	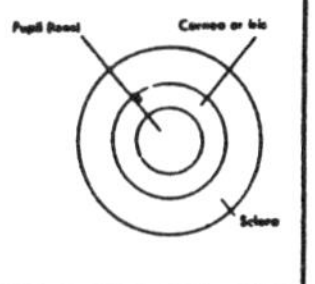
		2. LIDS:	A. DISTRICH	B. EPIPHORA	C. THIRD LID	D. INFECT.	
			E. MEBBOBIAN GL	F. TUMOR			
	(YES)	3. SCLERA:	A. INFECTED	B. HEMORRHAGIC	C. ICTERIC		
		4. CORNEA:	A. LACERATION	B. INFECTED	C. ULCER	D. EDEMA	
			E. VASCULARIZED	F. PERFORATED			
		5. CONJUNCTIVA:	A. HYPEREMIC	B. ICTERIC	C. PUSS	D. EDEMA	
		6. IRIS:	A. THICKENED	B. NON-RESPONS	C. DEFECT		
	NO	7. PUPILS:	A. DILATED	B. CONSTRICTED	C. UNEQUAL		
		8. LENS:	A. SCLEROTIC	B. CATARACT	C. LUXATED		
		9. FUNDUS:	A. OPTIC DISK	B. VESSELS	C. TAPATUM	D. NIGRUM	
			E. RETINA				
G. EARS		1. PINNA:	A. DROOPY	B. LACERATION	C. ALOPECIA	D. TUMOR	
	(YES)		E. INFLAMMED	F. INFECTED	G. HEMATOMA		
		2. CANAL:	A. INFLAMMED	B. INFECTED	C. WAX		
	NO		D. MITES	E. TUMOR			
		3. HEARING:	A. IMPAIRED	B. TOTAL DEAF			
H. CIRCULA-TION		1. CIRCULATION:	A. EDMIA	B. CYANOSIS	C. VENOUS >	D. SHOCK	
		2. MURMUR:	A. SYSTOLIC	B. DIASTOLIC	C. CONTINUOUS		
			D. MITRAL	E. TRICUSPID	F. AORTIC		
			G. PULMONIC	H. SEPTAL			
	(YES)		1. I 2. II 3. III 4. IV 5. V				
		3. RYHTHM:	A. SINUS CONTRACTIONS	B. BRADYCARDIA	C. TACHYCARD	D. PREMAT	
				E. ATRAL FIB	F. VENTRIC. FIB		
		4. PULSE:	A. WEAK	B. POUNDING	C. THREADY		
	NO	5. HEART SOUNDS:	A. MUFFLED	B. REFERRED	C. LOUDER RIGHT		
		6. VEINS:	A. > DISTENTION	B. < DISTENTION			
		7. CYANOSIS:	A. INTERMITTENT	B. CONSTANT			
		8. EDEMA	A. DEPENDENT	B. EXTREMITIES	C. HEAD/NECK		
I. ABDOMINAL		1. APPEARANCE:	A. PENDULOUS	B. DISTENDED	C. GAUNT	D. TENSE	
		2. ORGAN INVOLVED	A. STOMACH	B. LIVER	C. SPLEEN	D. S.I.	
	(YES)		E. L.I.	F. CECUM	G. COLON	H. KIDNEY	
			I. BLADDER	J. PROSPATE	K. L. NODE	L. UTERUS	
			M. OTHER________				
	NO		1. ENLARGED:	2. DISTENDED	3. MASS		
			4. SHRIVELED	5. SMALLER			
		3. HERNIA:	A. UMBLICAL	B. INGUINAL	C. PERINEAL	D. OTHER	
J. URO-GENITAL		1. WATER INTAKE:	A. INCREASED	B. DECREASED	C. NONE		
		2. URINE OUTPUT	A. INCREASED	B. DECREASED	C. NONE		
	(YES)	3. URINATION:	A. FREQUENT	B. BLOODY	C. INCONTIN	D. STRAIN	
		4. MALE:	A. PENIS	B. PREPUCE	C. TESTICLES		
			1. INFECTED	2. ENLARGED	3. UNDECENDED		
	NO	5. FEMALE:	A. VULVA	B. VAGINA			
			1. INFECTED	2. ENLARGED	3. TUMOR		
			C. LAST HEAT:________		D. LAST LITTER:________		
		6. BREASTS	A. ENLARGED	B. INFECTED	C. MASSES		
			D. NORMAL MILK	E. ABNOR. MILK	F. CYSTS		
K. NEURAL	(YES)	1. SIGNS:	A. HYPERESTHESIA	B. PARESIS	C. PARALYSIS		
	NO		D. SYNCOPE	E. SEIZURE	F. HEAD TILT		
			G. NYSTAGMUS	H. ATAXIA	I. COMMA		
L. LYMPH NODES	(YES)	1. ENLARGED:	A. MANDIBULAR	B. PRESCAPULAR	C. PREFEM	D. PELVIC	
	NO		E. ABDOMINAL	F. POPLITEAL	G. OTHER________		

Sample Computer Data form (page 2 of 2)

DATE ______________

DR. ______________

PROFESSIONAL SERVICES

1 WRITE IN
4 OFFICE VISIT/EXAM
7 PHYSICAL EXAM
10 OFFICE VISIT/EXAM
14 ABREVIATED EXAM
19 EMERG.OFFICE CALL
36 EXAM COURTESY
40 FOLLOW UP EXAM
44 HEALTH CERT.EXAM
90 O.V.SUT.REM.NO CHG
99 CLEAN ANAL SACS
104 BANDAGE SMALL
109 BAND.EAR POST-OP
116 CLEAN EARS COURTESY
118 FLUSH & MED. EARS
131 OPHTH-FLUORO STAIN
146 PEDICURE-COURTESY
147 PEDICURE-TECH

IMMUNIZATIONS

ADULT CANINE

3 ANNUAL PHYS EXAM
314 DHP ADULT/ANNUAL
363 CPV ADULT/ANNUAL
307 BORDETTELLA VAC W/ VAC

MESS.DHP 1 YR, CPV 3 WK - 3131

380 RABIES 1YR CANINE
384 RABIES 3YR CANINE

PUPPIES

5 NEW PUPPY EXAM
313 DHP (3WK)
361 CPV (3WK)

MESSAGE FECAL 3 WK - 31332

ADULT FELINE

3 ANNUAL PHYS EXAM
332 FVRCP ADULT/ANNUAL

MESSAGE FVRCP-FELV 1 YR -3321

349 FELEUK (1ST OF 2)
351 FELEUK ANNUAL

382 RABIES 1YR. FELINE
386 RABIES 3YR. FELINE

KITTENS

6 NEW KITTEN EXAM
331 FVRCP (3WK)
MESSAGE FECAL 3 WK - 31331

LABORATORY SERVICES

3100 WRITE IN
3103 GLUC CHEMSTRIP
3115 CYT.-ASPIRATION
3119 CYT.-EAR STAIN
3123 CYT.-SKIN SCRAPE

3133 FECAL FLOTATION
3135 FECAL 3 WK F.U.
3137 FECAL (ANNUAL)

3149 FELEUK - CITE
3151 FELEUK/FIV

3171 H.W. KNOTTS
3173 H.W. KNOTTS YRLY

3177 HEMATOCRIT (PCV)
3181 URINALYSIS COMPL

LAB COMMERCIAL

3200 WRITE IN
3203 COMPL PROFILE
3205 COMPL w/ NA & K
3207 PARTIAL PROFILE
3210 FEL. COMP. II

3276 COMPL. BLD CNT
3283 PLATELET COUNT

3303 CORTISOL-DEX&ACTH RESP MI
3304 CORTISOL-DEX OR ACTH RESP MI
3305 THYROID (T4) VDL
3306 THYROID FREE (T4)
3307 THYROID PROF MSU

3339 OCCULT HW VDL
3351 CULT. & SENS. VDL
3369 PAL PATH - SINGLE
3370 PAL LAB - MULTIPLE
3372 CYTOLOGY OSU

3381 ECG INITIAL

BOARDING SERVICES

5400 COURTESY - BTH

5401 DAY CARE
5405 BRD-CAN 1-25 LBS
5406 BRD-CAN 26-60 LBS
5407 BRD-CAN 61-90 LBS
5408 BRD-CAN >90 LBS
5410 BRD FELINE
5420 BRD-ADM.MED.QD
5421 BRD-ADM.MED.BID
5422 BRD-ADM.MED.TID
5430 SPEC DIET 1-25 LBS

INJECTIONS

1202 ALLERGY INJ.
1203 ACEPROM (MG)
1206 ACTH (IU)
1211 AMOXICILLIN INJ. (MG)
1216 ASPARGINASE-ELSPAR(IU)

1228 CAPARSOLATE (ML)
1231 CEFAZOLIN 1GM (VL)
1236 CHLORPROMAZINE (MG)
1237 CIMETIDINE (MG)

1247 DEPO MEDROL (MG)
1255 DEXAMETH.SOD.(ML)
1256 DEXAMETHASONE (ML)
1259 DEXTROSE 50% INJ(ML)
1261 DIAZEPAM (MG)

1271 DESOXYCORT-DOCP(MG)
1275 DOPRAM-V INJ (MG)
1290 EPOGEN INJ. (UNIT)
1297 GENTAMIC 50 MG/ML(ML)

1316 IVERMEC (MG)

1332 KETAM 100MG/ML (ML)

1336 LINCOCIN (ML)
1337 LIDOCAINE 2% (ML)

1347 MANNITOL 20% INJ (ML)
1349 METICORTEN 10MG (MG)
1350 METICORTEN 40 MG (MG)

1361 OXYTOCIN (ML)

1372 REGLAN (ML)

1400 TELAZOL (0.1 ML)
1403 TESTOST CYP. (MG)
1408 TORBUGESIC (MG)

1421 VETALOG 2MG/ML (MG)

FLUIDS

2007 DEX 5%.LRS
2017 DEX 5% IN WATER

2021 LRS

2025 SOD CHLORIDE 0.9%
2039 IV FL ADMIN.DISP.

Sample Computer Data form (page 1 of 2)

ANESTHESIA

HOSPITALIZATION

3800 WRITE IN
3806 HOSP. DAY CARE
3810 HOSP. (1-25 LBS.)
3811 HOSP. (26-60 LBS.)
3813 HOSP. (61-90 LBS.)
3815 HOSP. FELINE
3825 SPEC. DIET (1-25LBS)
3826 SPEC. DIET (26-60LBS)

3829 SPEC. DIET FELINE

PROFESSIONAL SERVICES HOSPITAL

3500 WRITE IN
3566 CATH.-IV (BTERFLY)
3567 CATH.-IV INDWEL
3637 EUTHANASIA COURTESY
3638 EUTHANASIA
3639 EUTH. W/ AFT CARE
3677 IN-PAT EVAL./CARE
3679 INTENSIVE CARE
3678 IN-PAT.EVAL./CARE

IN-PATIENT SERVICES

3900 WRITE IN
3911 ADMIN. MED. QD
3912 ADMIN. MED. BID
3913 ADMIN. MED. TID
4051 CATH. IV INDWEL
4121 SHAVE/SCRUB

RADIOLOGY

3400 WRITE IN
3495 RAD INTERP
3435 RAD-1 VW (14X17)
3436 RAD-2 VW (8X10)
3437 RAD-2 VW (10X12)
3438 RAD-2 VW (14X17)

3448 ADD VIEW (8X10)
3449 ADD VIEW (10X12)
3450 ADD VIEW (14X17)
3456 CONTRAST-DISPOSABLES
3459 CYSTO/URETH DISP
3473 ULTRASOUND THORAX
3477 ULTRASOUND ABDOMEN

DENTISTRY

5200 WRITE IN
5221 PROPHY/POL CAN
5220 POSTDENT PRPH EX
5297 DENTAL REMIND 1 YEAR
5296 DENTAL REMIND 6 MO

5222 PROPHY/POL FEL
5232 EXT INCISOR
5234 EXT PM (2 ROOT)
5236 EXT MOLAR

ANESTHESIA

5300 WRITE IN
5307 ANES PROPOFOL INJ (MG)
5308 PENTOTHAL 2.5% (ML)
5309 PENTOTHAL 5% (ML)
5312 HAL (1-10) .5H
5313 HAL (1-10) AD.25H
5314 HAL (11-25) .5H
5315 HAL (11-25) AD.25H
5316 HAL (26-60) .5H
5317 HAL (26-60) AD.25H
5318 HAL (61-100) .5H
5319 HAL (61-100) AD.25H
5329 ISO (1-10) .5HR
5330 ISO (1-10) AD.25H
5331 ISO (11-25) .5H
5332 ISO (11-25) AD .25H
5333 ISO (25-60) .5H
5334 ISO (25-60) AD.25H
5336 ISO (61-100) AD.25H

SURGERY

4200 WRITE IN
4270 NEUT-UPDATE MED. REC
4272 CAST.-CAN.(21-60)
4277 CAST.-FEL.
4321 DECLAW-FEL.
4620 OH UPDATE MED REC
4621 OVH (1-25)
4622 OVH (26-60)
4635 OVH-FELINE
4675 SKIN MASS (SMALL)

OPERATING ROOM AND SUPPLIES

4700 WRITE IN
4705 BASIC SURG PACK
4711 ELECTROCAUT PACK
4737 SURGERY DISPO.I
4739 SURGERY DISP. II

PRESCRIPTIONS AND HEARTWORM PREVENTATIVE

____
____
____
____
____
____

HEALTH AND MAINTENANCE SUPPLIES

____
____
____
____
____

PRESCRIPTION DIETS

____
____
____
____
____

MISCELLANEOUS, MESSAGES & RECALLS

4197 WEIGH PET #__________

____
____
____
____
____

Sample Computer Data form (page 2 of 2)

Patient: Lamb Chop Pat # 2A Sex : FS
Client : Krueger,Maxine

Breed: Poodle Wgt : 20
Birth : 04/21/85 Color : White

FVRCP: / / FeLV: / / FIP : / /
DHLP : 05/06/93 Lyme: 03/20/93 Rabies: 08/05/93
Fecal : 04/10/93 Dent: 06/26/93
HWT : 04/10/93 HWP: Heartgard
Medical Alert:

Patient Visitation Slip

Date	Patient No.
	Doctor No.
Appointment	Stored

DX | QTY

OFFICE VISITS/NEW CLIENTS

1 New Client Preparation
2 Office Visit Courtesy
3 Office Visit-routine

99 ____________

EXAMINATION SERVICES

100 After Hours Exam
101 Boarding Exam
102 Brief Exam
103 Comprehensive Exam
104 Consultation Services
105 Courtesy Exam
106 Emergency Exam
108 Health Certificate
110 Recheck Examination
111 Routine Examination
113 Exam w/Vaccines

199 ____________

PROFESSIONAL SERVICES/PROCEDURES

201 Anal Sac - expression
202 Anal Sac - infusion
204 Catheter - IV
205 Catheter - urinary
212 Cremation 15 lbs or less
213 Cremation 15 to 30 lbs
214 Cremation 30 to 60 lbs
215 Cremation 60 lbs & over
221 Euthanasia 15 lbs or less
222 Euthanasia 15 to 30 lbs
223 Euthanasia 30 to 60 lbs
224 Euthanasia 60 lbs & over
229 Fluid Thpy - IV/ml (O.P.)
230 Fluid Thpy - SC/ml (O.P.)
235 Office Inj.-analgesic
236 Office Inj.-antibiotic
237 Office Inj.-antidiarrheal
238 Office Inj.-antiemetic
239 Office Inj.-antipyretic
240 Office Inj.-diuretic
241 Office Inj.-hormone
242 Office Inj.-other
243 Office Inj.-sedation
244 Office Inj.-special
245 Office Inj.-steroid
246 Office Inj.-vitamin
247 Office Injection #1
248 Office Injection #2
249 Office Injection #3
250 Pedicure - Courtesy
251 Pedicure - Nail Trim

DX | QTY

270 Wound Care-clean/medicate

299 ____________

VACCINES

301 Bordetella Vaccination
303 Lyme Annual Vaccination
304 Lyme Vac Series #1
305 Lyme Vac Series #2
311 Parvovirus Vac
312 Parvo Vac (6 month)
321 Coronavirus Vaccination
334 DHLPP Annual Vac
335 DH-PP Puppy Vaccination
336 DHLPP Puppy Vac #1
337 DHLPP Puppy Vac #2
338 DHLPP Puppy Vac #3
340 Distemper/Measles Vac
355 FVRCP Annual Vac
356 FVRCP Kitten Vac #1
357 FVRCP Kitten Vac #2
358 FVRCP Kitten Vac #3
361 FeLV Annual Vac
362 FeLV Vac Series #1
363 FeLV Vac Series #2
365 FIP Annual Vac
366 FIP Vac Series #1
367 FIP Vac Series #2
372 Rabies Vac, Canine 1yr
373 Rabies Vac, Canine 3yr
374 Rabies Vac, Feline 1yr
375 Rabies Vac, Feline 3yr

399 ____________

LABORATORY SERVICES

406 BUN (azo-stix)
412 Glucose (sugar)
413 Glucose (stix-in house)
420 SMA Profile (major)
421 SMA Profile (minor)
439 CBC (complete blood count)
441 PCV (hematocrit)
462 Bacterial Culture (only)
463 Bact. Culture/Sensit'vty
464 Dermatophyte Culture
481 Ear Mite Swab
482 Fecal Exam (negative)
483 Fecal Exam (positive)
485 Heartworm Exam (negative)
486 Heartworm Exam (positive)
488 Skin Scraping (negative)
489 Skin Scraping (positive)
505 Histopathology
506 Histopathology (skin)

DX | QTY

507 Histopathology (special)
508 Necropsy Service 15# or less
509 Necropsy Service 15-30 lbs
510 Necropsy Service 30-60 lbs
511 Necropsy Service 60 lbs +
527 Brucellosis Titer
533 Feline Leuk.(IH) Test
534 Feline Leuk.(FA) Test
535 FIP Test
536 Immune Panel (complete)
540 Occult Heartworm Test
544 Thyroid Panel (complete)
559 Rabies Examination
562 Tissue Aspiration Fee
581 Urinalysis(complete)
583 Urinalysis (multi stix)
586 Urine Specific Gravity

599 ____________

RADIOLOGY

600 Add'l Radiograph(s)/films
601 Barium Administration
602 Consultation Services
603 GI(barium)Series, complete
604 GI (barium) Series, lower
605 GI (barium) Series, upper
606 Hip Dysplasia X-ray eval.
607 Interpretation/Hips OFA
608 Interpretation Fee
609 Postoperative Radiographs
610 Routine Radiographs

699 ____________

ANESTHESIA SERVICES

700 ECG Monitoring Service/hour
701 Gas/Inhalant-less than 15 lbs
702 Gas/Inhalant-15 to 30 lbs
703 Gas/Inhalant-30-60 lbs
704 Gas/Inhalant-60# or greater
705 Gen Gas/Inhalant Anesthesia
706 Intramuscular Inj.
707 Intravenous Inj.
708 Ketamine/Rompun Inj.
709 Ketamine/Valium Inj.
710 Local Anesthesia
711 Preanesthetic Inj.
712 Sedative Inj. - Rompun
713 Inhalation Therapy O_2/hour

799 ____________

Sample Computer Data form (page 1 of 2)

DX	SURGICAL SERVICES	QTY
	804 Bandaging Robert Jones	
	898 Declaw Feline (all)	
	899 Declaw Feline (front)	
	900 Declaw Feline (rear)	
	901 Declaw w/neutering	
	1123 Operating Room Fee	
	1124 Postoperative Care(major)	
	1125 Post-op Care (routine)	
	1126 Surgical Pack Fee	
	1127 Surgical Supply Fee	
	1144 Castration Abd. Crypt. X 1	
	1145 Castration Abd. Crypt. x 2	
	1146 Castration Inguinal Crypt.	
	1147 Cast. Inguinal Crypt. X 2	
	1148 Castration Routine - <15 #	
	1149 Castration Routine - 15-30	
	1150 Castration Routine - 30-60	
	1151 Castration Routine - 60# +	
	1152 Castration Routine, Feline	
	1153 Castration Scrotal Ablation	
	1154 Castration Testicular Tumor	
	1155 Castration Test. Tumor X 2	
	1171 OVH Comp., In Heat	
	1172 OVH Comp., Pregnant	
	1173 OVH Obese	
	1174 OVH Pyometra, Canine	
	1175 OVH Pyometra, Feline	
	1176 OVH Routine 15# or less	
	1177 OVH Routine - 15-30 lbs	
	1178 OVH Routine - 30-60 lbs	
	1179 OVH Routine - 60-90 lbs	
	1180 OVH Routine - 90 lbs +	
	1181 OVH Routine/Feline	
	1182 OVH Routine/In Heat	
	1183 OVH Routine/Pregnant	
	1184 OVH Tumor Removal	
	1194 Urinary Obstr./Feline	
	1199 ________________	
	HOSPITALIZATION SERVICES	
	1603 Fluid Thpy IV per ml	
	1604 Fluid Thpy SQ per ml	
	1621 Day Patient Care Only	
	1622 Intensive Care per day	
	1623 Observation Only per day	
	1624 Regular Daily Care 15# or <	
	1625 Regular Daily Care 15-30	
	1626 Regular Daily Care 30-60 lbs	
	1627 Regular Daily Care 60-90 lbs	
	1628 Regular Daily Care 90 lbs +	
	1699 ________________	

DX	GROOMING SERVICES	QTY
	2000 Bath and Dip 15 lbs or less	
	2001 15 to 30 lbs	
	2002 30 to 60 lbs	
	2003 60 to 90 lbs	
	2004 90 lbs or larger	
	2021 Ear Cleansing (routine)	
	2022 Ear Cleansing (severe)	
	2050 Mitaban B&D (mange tx)	
	2099 ________________	
	DENTAL	
	1800 Dental Cleaning (6 mos)	
	1801 Dental Cleaning-sev. 6 mo	
	1802 Dental Cleaning 12 mos	
	1803 Dental Cleaning-sev. 12 m	
	1804 Extraction(s) (complicated)	
	1805 Extraction(s) (routine)	
	1807 Polish Teeth (complicated)	
	1808 Polish Teeth (routine)	
	1899 ________________	
	BOARDING SERVICES	
	1901 Canine 15 lbs/day	
	1902 Canine 15 to 30 lbs/day	
	1903 Canine 30 to 60 lbs /day	
	1904 Canine 60 to 90 lbs /day	
	1905 Canine 90 + lbs /day	
	1906 Canine, nursing/day	
	1907 Feline Daily Boarding Fee	
	1908 Feline,nursing/day	
	1921 Day Care (only)	
	1922 Day Care (only) as Courtesy	
	1923 Exercise Boarder/day	
	1924 Isolation of Boarder/day	
	1925 Medicating Board./day (CA)	
	1926 Medicating Board./day (FE)	
	1999 ________________	
	DEWORMING	
	2100 Deworming-inject < 15 lbs	
	2101 Deworming-inject 15-30 lbs	
	2102 Deworming-inject 30-60 lbs	
	2103 Deworming-inject 60-90 lbs	
	2104 Deworming-inject 90 lbs or +	
	2105 Deworming-oral 15 lbs or <	
	2106 Deworming-oral 15-30 lbs	
	2107 Deworming-oral 30-60 lbs	
	2108 Deworming-oral 60-90 lbs	
	2109 Deworming-oral 90 lbs +	
	2199 ________________	

DX	PRESCRIPTIONS DISPENSED	QTY
	___-___-___ ___-___-___	
	___-___-___ ___-___-___	
	___-___-___ ___-___-___	
	___-___-___ ___-___-___	
	ADMINISTERED MEDICATIONS	
	___-___-___ ___-___-___	
	___-___-___ ___-___-___	
	___-___-___ ___-___-___	
	___-___-___ ___-___-___	
	PRESCRIPTION DIETS	
	___-___-___ ___-___-___	
	___-___-___ ___-___-___	
	___-___-___ ___-___-___	
	MISCELLANEOUS	
	5000 Patient Weight	

MESSAGE CODES

A100	Next Appointment
D1007	Obesity
D1028	Dental Tarter
D1665	HWT Disease Description
D1954	Flea Control
_____	________________
_____	________________
_____	________________
_____	________________
_____	________________

Sample Computer Data form (page 2 of 2)

```
                      COUNTY ANIMAL HOSPITAL OFFICE FORM

OWNER____________________________PET NAME______________ WEIGHT____________
PHONE NUMBER_____________________DOCTOR_________________TIME______________
A. PROBLEM/PROCEDURE CODE  (X=N/T  C/R=TREATED  O=TREATMENT NOT WANTED)

________ ________ ________ _________ _________ __________ _________ _____
B. PROFESSIONAL SERVICES C. VACCINATIONS     D. LABORATORY   E. HOSPITAL
1.  REGULAR (25)________ 1.DHLP-PV (1,2,3)   1.FECAL(____)   1.HOSP.K9(  )DAY
2.  FOLLOW-UP (20)______ 2.CR 3 YR_________  2.HW REG(___)   2.HOSP.FEL(  )DAY
3.  EMERGENCY (50)______ 3.FVRCP (1,2,3)__   3.HW OCC(___)   3.HOSP N/C(  )DAY
4.  CONSULT @___________ 4.FR 3 YR_________  4.CBC________   4.SPAY DOG (90)___
5.  NO CHARGE___________ 5.CVV (1,2,3)____   5.CHEMSCREEN_   5.SPAY CAT (80)___
6.  WELL VISIT (20)_____ 6.FD (1,2,3)_____   6.CS_________   6.CASTR DOG (75)__
7.  RE-CK.CONSULT@______ 7.FLV (1,2,3)____   7.UA_________   7.CASTR CAT (35)__
8.  PEDICURE (6)___(12)__ 8.CR 1 YR_________ 8.BUN________   8.DENT NO EXT_____
9.  EAR CLEANING (6)____ 9.FR 1 YR_________  9.BLGLUC_____   9.DENT EXTR.______
10. SCHIRMER TEAR_______ 10.BORD___________  10.THY_@______  10.ANESTH @_______
11. FLOUR.STAIN_________ 11.DHLP/PV/CVV___   11.FGL.CULT___  11.SURG_____@_____
12. INTRO OCUL.PRESS____                     12.BIOPSY@____  12.X-RAY_@________
13. EXT. OV (35)________                     13. __________  13.DECLAW(110)____
14. BANDAGE_____________ ******************  13. __________  14.TUMOR REM______
1A. HOUSE CALL (50)_____ B1C.NEW PET_____*   13. __________  29.ULTRASOUND_____
1B. PHONE CONSULT_______ ******************  14.SKIN SCRAPE  30.SHEL/CAT/SPAY__
-------------------------------------------  34.CYTOL@_____  31.SHEL/DOG/SPAY__
F.MISCELLANEOUS        11.GROOM/BATH_______  35.GRAM ST____  32.SHEL/CAT/CASTR_
1.EAR FLUSH(12)___     12.OTHER____________  36.TSH/STIM___  33.SHEL/DOG/CASTR_
2.PEDICURE(15)____     12.TECH.TIME___@____  37.ACTH/RES___  34.SPAY/DECLAW____
3.ANAL SACS(15)___     D.LABORATORY CON'T__  38.HI/DEX_____  35.SHEL/SPAY/DECLA
4.ECG (40)________     45.ANA                39.LO/DEX_____  36.SHEL/CASTR/DECL
5.REPEAT ECG(20)__     46.SERUM DIG          40.LYMES (20)_  36A.CASTR/DECLAW__
6.IV CATH(20)_____     47.SERUM PHENO        41.URINE PROFI  37.AURAL HEMAT@___
7.REPL.BANDAGE____     48.FELV ELISSA        42.COAG. (30)_  38. T.T.W.@_______
8.EUTH ONLY_______     49.FELV(HARDY)        43.PLATELETS    39.ABDCENTESIS____
9.EUTH&CREMA______     50.FELINE SEROLOGY    44.COOMBS(20)   40.THORACENT______
10.CREMATION______     51.BILE ACIDS (28)____ 45.ANA(20)___
G.INJECTIONS
DRUG  #  @  $   ml      DRUG   #  @   $   ml      DRUG   #   @   $   ml

____ ____ ___ ____      ____  ___ ___ ___         ____  ___   ____ _____

____ ____ ___ ____      ____  ___ ___ ___         ____  ___   ____ _____
____ ____ ___ ____      ____  ___ ___ ___         ____  ___   ____ _____
H.MEDICATIONS
DRUG   #     @          DRUG   #      @       DRUG       #        @
_____ ____ ________     _____ ____ _______    _____     ___   __________

_____ ____ ________     _____ ____ _______    _____     ___   ___________

_____ ____ ________     _____ ____ _______    _____     ___   ___________
I.RETURN VISIT          J.CALL BACK           K.RE-CHECK (CALL FOR APPT)
DATE      REASON        DATE     REASON       DATE     REASON
_____     ______        _____    _______      _____    _______
_____     ______        _____    _______      _____    ________
_____     ______        _____    _______      _____    ________
L.MESSAGES
1. OVERDUE DISTEMPER  2.OVERDUE RABIES  3.OVERDUE HW  4.HW TEST
5.STEROID  6.SKIN  7.DENTAL APPT.  8.HOSP.ANIMAL  9.NO SR.  10. NO EXEC.EXER
11.CALL NOT WELL  12.REMOVE BANDAGE  13. BANDAGE MGT  14. BANDAGE 7 DAYS
15.SR-1WK  16.SR-2WKS  17. REPL. LITTER  18.SPLINT/CAST  19  VOM/DIARR
20.WOUND/ABCESS  21.INT.PARASITES  22.EAR MED INSTR  23.URINE SPEC
24.STOOL SPEC   25.HW PREV INSTR  26. FLV CERT  27. CVV CERT  28.FERRET CERT
29.BORDETELLA  30.ESTIMATE  31.DHLP/PV/CVV CERT
M.CERTIFICATES: 47. HEALTH  48. FDV  49.DHLP/PV  50.RABIES

PAYMENTS: CHECK_____CASH_____M.C. _____VISA_____H.C. _____AMOUNT$__________
```

Sample Computer Data form

ANIMAL MEDICAL HOSPITAL
SCOTT G. WELLS, D.V.M.
55 SO. BLUFF ST.
ST. GEORGE, UTAH 84770
801 - 628-1634
Day or Night

CLIENT NAME ______________________ DIAGNOSIS CODE ____________

ANIMAL NAME ______________ FILE NO. ______________ REMINDER RECALL CODE ____________

Code	Item	FEE
10	**PROFESSIONAL EVALUATION**	
001	Office Visit	______
002	Initial Examination	______
003	Regular Examination	______
004	Multiple Examination	______
005	Comprehensive Examination	______
006	Geriatric Examination	______
007	Re-Examination	______
008	Health Certificate	______
009	EMERGENCY FEE	______
____	______________	______
20	**OUTPATIENT PROCEDURES**	
	PARASITE CONTROL	
001	Worm Small Dog	______
002	Worm Medium Dog	______
003	Worm Large Dog	______
004	Worm Cat	______
	HYPODERMIC INJECTIONS	
005	Antibiotics	______
006	Allergy Injection	______
007	Antiinflammatory	______
008	Analgesic	______
009	Abortion	______
010	Other Injections	______
011		______
	SPECIAL PROCEDURES	
012	Ear Cleaning Unilateral	______
013	Ear Cleaning Bilateral	______
014	Anal Sacs	______
015	Wound Preparation	______
016	Bandages/Wrap/Dressing Change	______
017	Casts and Splints	______
018	Nail Trim	______
019	Supplies	______
020	Special Procedures	______
____	______________	______
30	**ANESTHESIA/SURGERY**	
001	Premedication	______
002	General (Injections)	______
003	General (Injections & Inhalations)	______
004	Local	______
005	Sedation	______
006	Other	______
007	Pre-Surgical Exam	______
008	Operating Room	______
009	Surgical Pack General	______
010	Surgical Bone Pack	______
011	Extra Sponges & Suture	______
012	Penrose Drains	______
013	OHE Canine <20	______
014	OHE Canine 20 - 40	______
015	OHE Canine 40 - 60	______
016	OHE Canine 60 - 80	______
017	OHE Canine >80	______
018	OHE Pregnant	______
019	OHE Feline	______
020	Neuter Feline	______
021	Neuter Canine Small	______
022	Neuter Canine Medium	______
023	Neuter Canine Large	______
023	Cryptorchid Fee	______
025	Dewclaw Adult Canine	______
026	Declaw Feline	______
027	Declaw Feline & OHE	______
028	Declaw Feline & Neuter	______
029	SOFT TISSUE SURGERY	______
030	ORTHOPEDIC SURGERY	______
031	SPECIAL ORGAN SURGERY	______
032	Puppy T&D First	______
033	Puppy T&D Additional	______
034	Pin Removal	______
035	Cat Abscess Simple	______
036	Cat Abscess Complicated	______
037	Probe Foxtails & Foreign Obj	______
038	Surgical Assistant	______
039	Special Procedures	______
040	Supplies	______

Code	Item	Fee
40	**LABORATORY**	
001	Fecal Flotation	______
002	Fecal Direct	______
003	Urinalysis	______
004	Culture & Sensitivity	______
005	Pre-Anesthetic Profile	______
006	Heartworm	______
007	CBC Test Profile	______
008	Thyroid Profile	______
009	Glucose (Diabetes)	______
110	BUN Kidney	______
011	Chemistry Profile 1	______
012	Chemistry Profile 2	______
013	Needle Aspirate	______
014	Ear Mite Check	______
015	Allergy Testing	______
016	Leukemia Virus Test	______
017	Skin Scraping	______
018	Schirmer Tear Test	______
019	Flourescein Dye	______
020	Vaginal Smear	______
021	Histopathology (Biopsy)	______
022	Cytology	______
023	Laboratory Stain	______
024	Blood Draw &/or Urine Fee	______
025	Hemobartonellosis of FIP	______
026	Other	______
027	______________	______
____	______________	______
50	**RADIOLOGY**	
001	Survey Film & Interp 1 X-Ray	______
002	Survey Film & Interp 2 X-Rays	______
003	Additional Films	______
004	Special Studies & Interpret.	______
005	Certified Rad. Interpretation	______
006	Special Procedures	______
007	Supplies	______
____	______________	______
60	**PHARMACY**	
001	Dispensing Fee	______
002	Prescription Phone In	______
	All Prescriptions	
076	Other ______________	______
70	**IMMUNIZATIONS**	
001	Canine DHLPP (Parvo)	______
002	Feline Dist./Rhino/Calici	______
003	Feline Leukemia (FELV)	______
004	Rabies	______
005	Corona	______
006	Puppy DHLP - (Parvo)	______
007	Kitten FVRC	______
008	Kitten FELV	______
009	Puppy Plan	______
010	Kitten Plan	______
011	1 yr. Rabies	______
80	**DENTAL CARE**	
001	Pre-Dental Exam	______
002	Hand Scaling	______
003	Anesth & Ultrasonic Scaling Simple	______
004	Anesth & Scaling Complicated	______
005	Fluoride Treatment	______
006	Extractions	______
007	Special Procedures	______
008	Supplies	______
99	**HOSPITALIZATION & CARE**	
001	I.V. Catheters & Infusion Sets	______
002	I.V. Fluids 1st. Liter	______
003	I.V. Fluids Additional Liters	______
004	S.Q. Fluids	______
005	Blood Transfusion	______
006	Respiratory Therapy	______
007	Dr. Supervision & Nursing Care	______
008	Intensive Care	______
009	Hospitalization Large Patient	______
010	Hospitalization Small Patient	______
011	Hypodermic Injections	______
012	Oral Medications	______
013	Special Treatments	______
014	Other	______
____	______________	______

Code	Item	Fee
90	**PRESCRIPT. DIET & SCIENCE DIET**	
001	Feline C/D Case	______
002	Feline C/D 10lbs	______
003	Prescription/Can	______
004	Canine I/D Case	______
005	Canine I/D 10lbs	______
006	Canine R/D Case	______
007	Canine R/D 10lbs	______
008	Canine R/D 20lbs	______
009	Canine K/D Case	______
010	Canine Prescp/Can	______
011	Other	______
____	______________	______
11	**HOSPITAL SPECIAL SERV**	
001	Boarding Small/Day	______
002	Boarding Small Multi/Day	______
003	Boarding Large/Day	______
004	Boarding Large Multi/Day	______
005	Bath Non Medicated Small	______
006	Bath Non Med Extra Fee	______
007	Bath Medicated Small	______
008	Bath Medicated Extra Fee	______
009	Euthanasia Small	______
010	Euthanasia Large	______
011	Burial Small	______
012	Burial Large	______
013	Euthansia with Sedation	______
014	Other	______
____	______________	______
12	**NON-PRESCRIPTION ITEMS**	
____	Vitamins	______
____	Flea/Tick/Etc.	______
____	Other Supplies	______
001	Pet Tabs 60	______
002	Pet Tabs 180	______
003	Derm Caps Reg.	______
004	Derm Caps ES	______
005	Mycodex Shampoo	______
006	Pearlescent Shampoo	______
007	Mycodex Flea & Tick Spray	______
008	Flea & Tick Medication	______
009	Eliminodor	______
010	Nutrical	______
011	Cat & Dog Laxative	______
012	Other ______________	______

Estimates and fees may vary according to the degree of difficulty in establishing a diagnosis and your pets response to treatment.

Estimate ______________ To ______________

TOTAL CHARGES	______
DEPOSIT	______
BALANCE DUE	______

CASH	CK	MC	VISA	INITIAL:

HOME CARE INSTRUCTIONS:

____
____
____
____
____

reprinted with permission of Ancom Business Products 800/845-9010

Sample Computer Data form

CREDIT AGREEMENT

Name of Client: ______________________________

Address: ______________________________

Employer: ____________________ SS#: ____________

Work Phone: ____________________ Home Phone: ____________

1) Amount of unpaid professional fees: $ ____________

2) Credit Service Fee: $ ____________

3) Total amount financed: $ ____________

TERMS:

Each of the below monthly payments is due on expected by the ___th of the month. If payment is not received at the above office in 15 days, a $10.00 LATE PAYMENT CHARGE will be added to the account.

INTEREST:

18% per year (1 1/2% per month) of the unpaid balance of the amount financed and late charges that may apply.

For the first 90 days, this is included int he Credit Service Fee. After 90 days, interest (at the rate of 1 1/2% per month) will be added to the account.

AGREEMENT:

1) Monthly Payment . . . . $ ____________

2) Final Payment . . . . . $ ____________

3) Plus any Late Charges or interest that may apply.

I agree to make the first monthly payment the ___th of __________, 19___, and subsequent payments each month until paid in full. I have read the above, agree to the terms and interest rate, and have received a copy of the agreement.

____________________ ______________________________

Date Signature of Client

Sample Credit Agreement form

PAYMENT AGREEMENT

Date: ______________________ Owner: ______________________

Phone: ______________________ Animal Name: ______________________

Mailing Address: ____

____

Agreement:

Owner hereby agrees to pay ABC Veterinary Hospital in __________ monthly installment(s) of $______________________. The first installment being due on the ________ day of ______________. All the remaining installments will be due on the same day of each consecutive month until paid in full.

Charges:

Late payment charge - There will be no late payment charge assessed if payments are made on time. A 10% late payment charge will be assessed ($1.00 minimum, $15.00 maximum) on each payment not paid within 10 days of payment due date.

Returned Check Charge - There will be a $10.00 charge when a check submitted by you for payment is returned to the bank for insufficient funds.

I HEREBY CERTIFY that I have read and received a copy of the aforegoing payment agreement and further, understand its terms and declarations.

______________________________________ DATE ______________

Signature of Owner
or parent if owner is a minor

____

Staff Initials

Sample Payment Agreement form

THIRD PARTY AUTHORIZATION

Dear ______________________________:

One of our clients, ____, has informed us that you will assume financial responsibility for veterinary services the client is currently receiving from ______ (hospital/clinic name)______________. In order to verify this, we would like you to sign and return the following authorization form.

Yours truly,

____

I, the undersigned, do promise to pay for the __(type)__________ serviced rendered by ____, D.V.M. to ______(Pet's Name)__________.

____________________ ________________________________

Date of Signature Signature

Sample Third Party Authorization form

PROMISSORY NOTE

$________________________ Date: __________________________

FOR SERVICES RECEIVED, the undersigned promises to pay to ABC Animal Clinic the principal sum of $ ______________________, by _________________________________. After this date interest will be charged (1 1/2% per month) at the rate of 18 percent per annum. If payment is not received in full, including interest, 30 days from agreed date, the account will be turned over for collection.

DATED at ____________ the _________ day of __________________, 199__.

Client Signature: ____

Address____

Telephone No. _______________________ SS #: __________________

Employer ____

Employer Address: ____

Employer Telephone No.: ______________________________________

Reference: ____________________ Relationship: ________________

Address: ____

Telephone No.: ____

Sample Promissory Note form

Appendix E

FINANCIAL STATEMENTS AND GLOSSARY

Table 2-1
Balance Sheet

Cedarton Animal Hospital, Inc.
Statement of Assets and Liabilities
December 31, 1986
Cash Basis

ASSETS		
CURRENT ASSETS		
Cash		
Petty cash-imprest	$ 150	
Checking account	5,000	
Bank money-market funds	10,000	
(Accounts receivable)*	(0)	
Notes receivable from officers	1,000	
Drugs & medical supply inventory	3,600	
Total current assets		$19,750
PROPERTY AND EQUIPMENT		
Medical equipment	24,055	
Accumulated depreciation	(8,840)	
Office equipment, furniture, & fixtures	12,500	
Accumulated depreciation	(9,540)	
Practice vehicles	0	
Accumulated depreciation	(0)	
Leasehold improvements	12,275	
Accumulated depreciation	(1,875)	
Buildings	0	
Accumulated depreciation	(0)	
Net property and equipment	28,575	
TOTAL ASSETS		$48,325
LIABILITIES & SHAREHOLDER EQUITY		
CURRENT LIABILITIES		
Short-term notes, loans, & advances	$ 5,500	
(Accounts payable)*	(0)	
Accrued liabilities		
Federal income tax & FICA withholdings	1,935	
State income tax withholdings	480	
Accrued profit-sharing plan	(0)	
Total current liabilities		7,915
LONG-TERM LIABILITIES		
Long-term debt	13,200	
Total long-term liabilities		13,200
TOTAL LIABILITIES		21,115
SHAREHOLDERS EQUITY		
Common stock	10,000	
Retained earnings	17,210	
Total shareholders equity		27,210
TOTAL LIABILITIES & SHAREHOLDERS EQUITY		$48,325

* In Cash Basis balance sheets prepared for creditors, a conversion often is made to accrual reporting. As a result, accounts receivable, accounts payable, and any other significant assets or liabilities would be stated. For these reasons, the balance sheet frequently is a "hybridized" combination of cash and accrual forms.

Reprinted from *Successful Financial Management for the Veterinary Practice* by Robert Froehlich, DVM, MBA

Sample Balance Sheet

Table 2-3
"Income Statement"

Cedarton Animal Hospital
Statement of Revenues and Expenses
For 12 Months Ending December 31, 1986

	Current	%	Year to Date	%
INCOME FROM OPERATIONS				
Fees for services*	$28,550	91.9	$291,876	90.8
Ancillary companion animal services	2,506	8.1	29,632	9.2
Total income from operations	31,056	100.0	321,508	100.0
COST OF PROFESSIONAL SERVICES				
Drugs & medical supplies	2,490	8.0	28,614	8.9
Laboratory costs	785	2.5	8,035	2.5
Ancillary companion animal services costs	930	3.0	12,539	3.9
GENERAL & ADMINISTRATIVE EXPENSES				
Compensation of veterinary officers	6,385	20.6	108,600	33.8
Other salaries & wages	5,930	19.0	58,514	18.2
Payroll taxes	862	2.8	9,458	2.9
Sales and use tax	170	0.5	1,335	0.4
Profit-sharing plan	5,530	17.8	5,530	1.7
Laundry and uniforms	155	0.5	1,150	0.4
Continuing education	0	0	3,000	0.9
Rent on business property	2,100	6.8	25,400	7.9
Maintenance/service contracts	280	0.9	5,450	1.7
Insurance	0	0	5,785	1.8
Real estate tax	2,650	8.5	2,650	0.8
Personal property tax	0	0	610	0.2
Utilities	650	2.1	3,400	1.1
Telephone	435	1.4	3,398	1.1
Advertising and promotion	1,265	4.2	8,248	2.5
Office supplies	685	2.5	3,510	1.1
Postage expense	355	1.1	1,925	0.6
Accounting services	780	2.5	3,820	1.2
Depreciation	745	2.4	6,970	2.2
Interest expense	61	0.2	1,540	0.5
Total expense	33,243	107.0	309,481	96.3
Income from operations	(2,187)	(7.0)	12,027	3.7
Other income (expense)	55	0.2	720	0.1
Income before taxes	(2,132)	(6.9)	12,747	3.9
Less income tax provisions	0	0	2,675	0.8
Net income			$ 10,072	3.1

* Although further division of income by source may be desired (*eg*—pharmacy, surgery, etc.), it is shown here in one category for ease of illustration.

Note: Column totals may not equal 100% because of rounding off figures.

Reprinted from *Successful Financial Management for the Veterinary Practice* by Robert Froehlich, DVM, MBA

Sample Income Statement

Glossary of Accounting Terms

reprinted from Successful Financial Management for the Veterinary Practice by Robert Froehlich, DVM, MBA

Accelerated depreciation Any method of calculating depreciation which results in larger depreciation deductions in the early years of the asset's life. Examples are double declining balance and sum-of-the-years' digits methods.

Account A segment of the ledger in which increases and decreases are accumulated for individual assets, liabilities, equities, revenues, and expenses. The listing of account titles is called a chart of accounts.

Accountability The capability and responsibility to account for the expenditure of money and commitment of other resources in terms of the results achieved. This involves both the stewardship of money and other capital resources and the evaluation of achievement in relation to specified goals.

Accounting 1) The procedure of maintaining systematic records, largely financial in nature, and summarizing, analyzing, and interpreting the results of such records. 2) The communication of economic data, largely financial, useful to decision makers.

Accounting cycle The sequence of accounting procedures starting with journal entries and ending with financial statements.

Accounting period A time period at the end of which, and for which, financial statements are prepared for the practice; for example, January 1 to December 31. (See fiscal period.)

Accounting principles The principles that explain current accounting concepts and practices and that guide in the selection among alternative treatments for reporting transactions.

Accounting system The total mechanism of records and procedures of recording, retrieving, and reporting information on the financial position and operations of the practice.

Accounts payable The liabilities on open account owed by the practice to outside persons or entities for goods and services received.

Accounts receivable An open account of amounts owed to the practice by outside persons or entities, usually clients, for goods and services furnished by the practice.

Accrual basis of accounting A basis of accounting that identifies revenues with the period in which service is provided (to generate the revenues) regardless of when cash is received and that identifies expenses with the period in which resources are consumed (to generate the revenues) regardless of when cash is paid. Because revenues and expenses are easier to predict on the accrual basis, accrual accounting is normally used to prepare operating budgets.

Accumulated depreciation A preferred title for the contra account that shows the total of depreciation recorded for an asset since it was acquired. Older and less acceptable terms are allowance for depreciation or reserve for depreciation.

Acid test ratio The sum of cash, marketable securities, and current receivables divided by current liabilities. Often called the quick asset ratio or liquidity ratio, it is used in assessing relative liquidity of the practice. Because of the omission of several assets and liabilities from the cash-basis position statement, this ration should be applied only to the accrual-basis position statement.

Additional paid-in capital Another title for capital contributed in excess of par (or stated) value for practices organized as corporations.

Adjusted basis The basis used to compute gain or loss on disposition of an asset for tax purposes.

Administrative expense An expense incurred for the practice as a whole as contrasted to an expense incurred for a more specific function.

Aging patient receivables A method of reviewing and classifying patient receivables by the time elapsed (usually in number of months) since the receivables came into existence, for the purpose of evaluating credit and collection policies and estimating the amount of uncollectible accounts receivable as of a given date.

Amortization The general process of allocating the acquisition costs of assets to the periods of benefit; called depreciation for plant assets, depletion for wasting assets (natural resources), and amortization for intangible assets.

Annual report A report for stockholders and other interested parties prepared for the fiscal year; includes a statement of financial position, an income statement, a statement of changes in financial position, the auditor's report, and perhaps comments from management about the year's events.

Annuity An amount payable yearly or at other regular intervals. A series of equal payments at equally spaced time intervals.

Appraisal The act of making an estimate of value, particularly of the value of property, by systematic procedures that include physical examination, pricing, and often engineering estimates. Also, the value established by estimating.

Arm's length transaction A transaction negotiated by unrelated parties, each acting in his or her own self-interest.

Articles of incorporation A legal document filed with state authorities by persons forming a corporation. When the document is returned with a certificate of incorporation, it becomes the corporation's charter. (See charter.)

Assessed valuation A valuation set upon real estate or other property by a taxing authority as the basis for levying taxes.

Assessment, special A compulsory levy made by a local government on certain properties to defray part or all of the cost of a specific improvement or service that is presumed to be of general benefit to the public and of special benefit to the owners of such properties.

Assets The resources controlled by the practice.

Audit The examination of records and documents and the securing of other evidence for one or more of the following purposes: 1) determining the propriety (legality) of proposed or completed transactions, 2) ascertaining whether all transactions have been recorded, 3) determining whether transactions are accurately recorded in the accounts and in the statements drawn from the accounts, and 4) satisfying generally accepted auditing standards so that an independent auditor may express an opinion as to the fairness of the financial statements.

Auditor An official or accountant authorized to examine financial accounts for accuracy.

Auditor's report The auditor's statement of the work he has done and his opinion on the fairness of the financial statements.

Audit trail The set of references in an accounting system that allows an accounting event to be traced from original documents through the accounting system into the financial statements.

Authorized capital stock The number of shares of stock that can be issued by a corporation, as specified in the articles of incorporation.

Average cost Fixed costs plus variable costs (total costs) divided by the units produced or units of service rendered.

Bad debt An uncollectible account receivable.

Bad debt policy 1) The decision rules that recognize bad debt expense and corresponding reduction in the carrying value of total accounts receivable prior to identifying specific uncollectible accounts. 2) It also includes guides as to when specific receivables are written off the accounts.

Balance sheet 1) A summary of the financial status of the practice with an accounting of all assets and liabilities at a given date. 2) A statement on the accrual basis of the financial position of the practice, as of a given date, showing assets, liabilities, and equity. Also called statement of financial position.

Bank reconciliation statement A statement that explains the difference between the balance of the cash in the bank account as shown on the practice's books and the balance on the bank statement; it also provides a corrected balance of cash in bank for the practice's records. It takes into account the amount of such items as checks issued that have not cleared or deposits made that have not been recorded by the bank, as well as errors made by the bank or the practice.

Bank statement A statement sent by the bank to checking account customers showing deposits, checks cleared, and service charges for a period of usually one month.

Betterment An addition made to, or change made in, a fixed asset that is expected to prolong its life or increase its efficiency over and above routine maintenance; the cost of the betterment therefore is added to the book value of the asset.

Bill A statement of account submitted to a patient.

Bonus A premium over normal wage or salary paid to employees, usually for meritorious performance.

Booking The recording of charges in preparation for billing.

Bookkeeping The process of analyzing and recording transactions in the accounting records.

Book loss The loss recorded in the operating statement of the practice when a capitalized asset is sold for less than its book value.

Book value The amount at which a given resource is carried in the financial records of the practice: conventional accounting methods require the use of historical cost. It does not necessarily have any relationship to fair market value.

Break-even chart A graphic presentation of the interaction of revenues and costs at varying volumes of activity (number of patients).

Break-even point The activity level where total revenues equal total costs. Graphically, the break-even point is where the total revenues line intersects the total costs line. The break-even point may be expressed in units of service or in dollars of revenue.

Budget An expression of the practice's operational plan, in dollars and cents, over a specific period of time. The budget serves as a basis for determining the practice's financial ability to attain predetermined goals and for evaluating operating performance. Also called a profit plan.

Budget variance The difference between the actual costs incurred and the budget, adjusted to actual activity level.

Bylaws The rules adopted by the stockholders of a corporation that specify the general methods for carrying out the functions of the corporation.

Capital asset An asset whose benefit is to be used over a long period of time rather than in the period of acquisition. Property such as equipment or buildings, whose cost is depreciated over an economic life.

Capital budgeting The planning and decision process where a determination is made on how to best utilize the financial resources available to a business. Considerations include alternative investment projects, fixed equipment and assets, capital costs, and return on the funds invested.

Capital expenditures The amounts paid for the acquisition of fixed assets or additions to fixed assets that are presumed to provide benefits for more than one year. Amounts expended for land or existing buildings, improvements of grounds, construction of buildings, additions to buildings, remodeling of buildings, and replacement of equipment are all examples of capital expenditures.

Capital expenditures budget The portion of a practice's comprehensive budget that relates to the procurement or disposition of long-lived productive resources.

Capital gain or loss Gain or loss on the sale of assets that are not held for resale as inventory and have been owned by the practice for a minimum period of time (usually one year). A capital gain had formerly been taxed at a lower rate than ordinary income.

Capital stock The ownership shares of a corporation; consists of common and preferred stock.

Capital structure The composition of a corporation's equities; the relative proportions of short-term debt, long-term debt, and owners' equity.

Cash basis of accounting A basis of accounting that recognizes revenues only in the accounting period when cash is collected and expenses only in the accounting period when cash is paid.

Cash budget A projected breakdown of cash receipts and other inflows as well as expenses and other outflows projected over a period (such as a year) and divided into activity periods (such as months).

Cash flow The sum of net income plus depreciation. Cash flow recognizes the real dollars available for spending during a given period of financial activity.

Charges The full price of services provided patients.

Charter A grant of rights from the state to a business corporation, such as the right to incorporate and transact business.

Chart of accounts The listing of all the titles and respective numbers of all accounts in the general ledger which categorizes all the flows of cash and lists all the debts and assets of the business.

Collection cycle (period) The average period of time from when a service is performed and the patient is billed to when payment is collected for the service.

Collection policy The protocols established which determine a follow-up on slow-paying accounts.

Common stock The stock representing the veterinary practice owners who have a residual claim on the assets and earnings of the practice after all debts and preferred stockholders' claims have been met.

Comparative statements Financial statements showing information for the same practice for different time periods, usually for two successive years.

Compensating balance The amount a bank requires a commercial customer to maintain on deposit in the customer's checking account as a condition for a loan. The balance usually is expressed as a percentage of the loan and increases the effective interest rate.

Compound interest The interest calculated on principal plus previously undistributed interest.

Comprehensive budget The budget that consolidates the practice's overall operating plans. It includes the cash budget, the operating budget (profit plan), and the projected statement of financial position. Also called the master budget.

Conservatism An accounting concept that calls for recognition of all losses and expenses as soon as possible but defers recognition of gains or profits until they are realized through a market transaction or exchange.

Constraint A restriction on the business's operations limiting the amount of resources that can be committed to a project, service, or activity. Often imposed by bank of debt holder, e.g., bondholder.

Contingent liabilities Items that may become liabilities as a result of conditions undetermined at a given date, such as pending lawsuits, judgments under appeal, and unsettled disputed claims.

Contra account An account, such as accumulated depreciation, that accumulates subtractions from another account, such as buildings.

Contract A binding promissory agreement between two or more parties.

Contracted services The services rendered to the practice by persons who are not on the payroll of the practice, including all related expenses covered by the contract.

Control The process of monitoring, measuring, and correcting actual performance to ensure that the practice's goals and objectives are accomplished.

Controllable cost A cost that can be influenced by a manager in either the short run or the long run. A cost that is the responsibility of a specific manager.

Controller A business's principal accounting officer responsible for planning and controlling the organization's financial database.

Corporation An organization formed for legal and tax purposes that is recognized as a separate and distinct entity.

Cost The consideration given to acquire a resource. It is measured by the cash paid for the resource or the cash equivalent of the resource, whichever can be measured most objectively.

Cost accounting The body of accounting that provides for the assembling and recording of all the elements of cost incurred to accomplish a purpose, to carry on an activity or operation, or to complete a unit of work or a specific job.

Cost-benefit analysis The comparison of the cost of a program with its expected benefits, expressed in dollars. Also called benefit-cost analysis.

Cost center In cost accounting, a responsibility center that does not serve patients directly and to which only costs may be traced.

Cost effectiveness analysis An analysis of the relationship between the benefits, expressed in nonfinancial terms, and the dollar costs of a particular project or activity.

Cost of capital The cost of providing financial resources for the practice, including interest on debt and cost of maintaining adequate owners' equity.

Credit period The length of time that credit is granted.

Credit standards The criteria a business uses for granting of credit to a client.

Current assets Cash and other assets that are expected to be converted to cash in the normal course of operations or within one year.

Current liabilities Liabilities that will mature and require payment from current assets within one year.

Current ratio Current assets divided by current liabilities; used as a measure of the liquidity of a practice.

Database Information available to a practice for planning, decision making, and control functions.

Debt ratio The ratio of long-term debt to capital structure. (It is sometimes computed as the ratio of total debt to total assets.) The debt ratio shows relative risk of creditors and owners.

Debt service Expenditures for the retirement of noncurrent or long-term debt, including principal and interest on such debt.

Declining-balance depreciation The method of calculating the periodic deprecation charge by multiplying the undepreciated cost (net book value) at the beginning of the period by a constant percentage.

Deficit A debit balance in the retained earnings account.

Demand note A promissory note expressly stating that the principal is payable on demand.

Depreciation The process of allocating the original cost of a capital asset in a systematic and rational manner over the useful life of the asset. On an income statement, the noncash expense which, for accounting purposes, adjust the value of a fixed asset due to wear and tear and the passage of time.

Direct expenses Costs that are directly attributable to a specific cost objective, such as a cost center, and are traceable to that cost objective.

Discount rate The interest rate used to discount future cash flows to their present value.

Discounted cash flow Any capital investment decision technique that adjusts cash flows over the life of the investment for the time value of money.

Discretionary cost Fixed costs that arise from specific management decisions to use a specific amount of a resource. Also called programmed costs.

Dividend A distribution of earnings to owners of a corporation payable in cash, shares of stock, or property. Dividends, except stock dividends, become a legal liability of the corporation when they are declared.

Double entry A system of accounting that recognizes that for every transaction equivalent debit and credit entries are made.

Earnings Net income (sometimes called profit).

Earnings per share Net income divided by number of shares outstanding.

Economic order quantity(EOQ) In materials management, the optimal amount of supplies to order when the inventory is reduced to a level called the reorder point.

Economy of scale The theoretical cost savings resulting from aggregation of resources in the larger practice.

Employee benefits Amounts paid by the practice on behalf of employees that are not included in their gross salary. Such payments are usually considered overhead expenses and, while not paid directly to employees, nevertheless are part of the cost of employee compensation. Examples are 1) group health and life insurance policies, 2) contributions to employee retirement programs, 3) education allowances, and 4) paid vacations. Also called fringe benefits.

Entity A person, partnership, corporation, or other organization for which accounting records are maintained.

Entry The record of a financial transaction in its appropriate book of account.

Equities Liabilities plus owners' equity.

Equity Equity is the excess of assets over liabilities. Normally this excess is called owners' equity or stockholders' equity.

Equity ratio Owners' equity divided by total assets.

Expense account A ledger account used to accumulate expenses; such accounts are closed at the end of the accounting period.

External reporting Reporting of financial activities and status to parties outside the practice, as opposed to internal reporting for the benefit of management.

Extraordinary item A material gain or loss item characterized both by its *unusual nature and the likelihood that it will not reoccur*, given the nature of the environment in which the practice operates. It is shown, along with its income tax effects, separately from income from continuing operations on the income statement.

Factoring The practice of selling accounts receivable to a collection agent at a discount.

Fair market value The value of assets as established by what a willing buyer will pay to a willing seller in the open market at a given time.

Fee-for-service 1) A charge set for a type of service rendered. 2) The method of paying for care that assigns individual service charges to patients and involves retrospective reimbursement only for the services actually rendered, as distinct from "prepayment" or "prospective payment."

Fee schedule A listing of a practice's charges for specific procedures.

Financial accounting The body of accounting concerned with preparation of general purpose financial statements for the owner(s) of the practice and external reporting. It is to be distinguished from management accounting.

Financial statements The general purpose reports on the stewardship of the practice prepared for management and external purposes. They include a statement showing financial position, a statement showing the results of operations for the period, and a statement showing sources and uses of funds. Financial statements may be prepared either on the cash or accrual basis.

Fiscal period Any accounting period at the end of which a practice determines its financial position and the results of its operations and closes its books. It is usually a year, though not necessarily a calendar year. The most common fiscal period for animal hospitals is January 1 through December 31. (See accounting period.)

Fixed assets Long-lived tangible assets used in the operation of the practice. Land, buildings, equipment, and furniture in current use.

Fixed costs Costs that are incurred regardless of the volume of service and that do not vary with changes in activity; as distinct from variable costs. Also called constant costs.

Fixed liability A long-term liability (maturity beyond one year) of the practice.

Flexible budget A statement of how costs change with changes in activity, such as a change in the number of patient visits; often expressed as the formula for total costs, TC = FC + VC (X) where FC is the fixed costs, VC is the variable cost, and X is a measure of activity level.

Forecast A projection that is used in the development of plans and budgets.

Fringe benefits Benefits, other than wages or salaries, provided by an employer for employees. Examples are health insurance, vacation time, and disability income. Also called employee benefits.

Full-time equivalent (FTE) The amount of employee or professional time expressed in proportion to the time required in a full-time position, with "1.0" representing one full-time position. The number of full-time equivalent employees in a practice is usually expressed in absolute terms, such as 8.5 FTE employees.

Funded Said of a pension plan, construction fund, or other obligation when funds have been set aside for meeting the obligation when it becomes due.

Funds statement A name formerly used for the statement of changes in financial position.

Future value (FV) The amount to which a payment or series of payments will grow at a stated future date when compounded by a given interest rate.

Gain Excess of consideration received over book value from a specific transaction.

General ledger A book, file, or other device in which accounts are kept to the degree of detail necessary and that summarizes the financial transactions of the practice. (See ledger.)

General partner A member of a partnership who normally will participate in the management of the partnership and who has unlimited liability for all debts of the partnership; in contrast with a limited partner.

Generally accepted accounting principles (GAAP) As defined by the Accounting Principles Board and the Financial Accounting Standards Board of the AICPA, the conventions, rules and procedures necessary to define accepted accounting practice at a particular time; includes both broad guidelines and relatively detailed practices and procedures.

Goal A broad statement of the direction toward which all decisions and activities of a clinic are focused.

Going concern assumption For accounting purposes, a practice is assumed to remain in operation long enough for all its current plans to be carried out.

Goodwill The excess of cost paid for an acquired firm or operating unit over the current value of the net assets of the acquired unit. Informally used to indicate value expressed in dollars of good customer relations, high employee morale, a well-respected business name, and so on, which intangible assets are expected to result in greater than normal earning power.

Gross income Total revenues before deducting any expenses; an expression employed in the accounting for individuals, financial institutions, and the like.

Group practice A practice formally organized to provide veterinary care through the services of three or more veterinarians, using office space, equipment, and/or support personnel jointly.

Group insurance Insurance covering a group of persons, usually employees of a single employer or members of a union local, under one contract for the benefit of the members of the group.

Imprest fund A petty cash fund that is reimbursed periodically for the amount expended from the fund.

Income Excess of revenues earned over expenses incurred in carrying on the practice's operations. It should not be used without an appropriate modifier such as operating, nonoperating, or net. Note: The term income should not be used in lieu of revenues.

Income statement A statement that evaluates operating performance by comparing revenues (accomplishments) with expired costs (efforts); accrual-basis operating statement.

Indirect expenses Those elements of cost necessary in the provision of a service that are of such a nature that they cannot be readily or accurately identified with or traced to the specific service, for example, heat, electricity, office space, administration. (See overhead.)

Information system An organized structure to provide information to facilitate decision making, planning, control, and reporting.

Intangible property A nonphysical, noncurrent asset with future benefit; such as a patent, goodwill.

Interest A fee charged a borrower for the use of money. (See debt service.)

Internal control A plan of organization under which employees' duties are so arranged, and records and procedures so designed, as to make it possible to exercise effective accounting control over assets, liabilities, revenues, and expenditures. For example, under such a system the employees' work is subdivided so that no one employee performs a complete cycle of operations; an employee handling cash would not post the accounts receivable records. Under such a system, the procedures to be followed are stated and proper authorization is required for all actions to be taken.

Inventory The cost of supplies and equipment in storage awaiting use.

Investment tax credit A special tax provision that allows direct reductions of income taxes for the acquisition of certain depreciable assets.

Invoice An itemized statement of goods or services provided to a customer.

Journal Any form in which the financial transactions of the practice are formally recorded for the first time, such as the cash receipts book, check register, and general journal.

Keogh Act plan A formal retirement plan available since 1963 to self-employed individuals and nonincorporated partnerships.

Land account A fixed asset account that reflects the acquisition value of land owned by a practice. If land is purchased, this account includes the purchase price and costs such as legal fees, filing and excavation costs, and other associated improvement costs that are incurred to put the land in condition for its intended use.

Lease A contract used in the rental of buildings and capital equipment.

Ledger A group of accounts in which the financial transactions of a practice are recorded. (See general ledger.)

Lessee User of leased assets.

Lessor Owner of leased assets.

Liabilities An obligation arising out of past events or transactions payable in cash or other resources usually at some specified or determinable date in the future.

Limited partner A member of a partnership normally with management participation whose exposure to liability is limited to the extent of investment, in contrast with a general partner.

Liquidating dividend A dividend declared in the winding up of a corporation to distribute the assets of the practice to the stockholders.

Liquidity The amount and composition of a practice's assets with emphasis upon their conversion to cash.

Log book A department record of services rendered, which readily identifies procedures with individual patients.

Long-range decisions Decisions adding to or reducing the productive capability of a practice. These decisions affect the cash flows of more than one accounting period so that the time value of money is a significant variable.

Loss The cost of a resource that has been consumed without providing a benefit or revenue.

Management accounting The body of accounting that focuses on the information needs of management for planning and controlling the practice's operations, as distinguished from financial accounting.

Management by exception The focus of attention only on those activities where actual performance differs significantly from planned performance.

Management control The process of monitoring the productivity and utilization practices of responsibility centers within the organization and instituting changes beneficial to the practice as a whole.

Management information system A network of communication channels that acquires, retrieves, and redistributes data used in managing the practice in and supporting the individual and collective decision-making processes.

Matching The accounting process of relating costs and revenues in the determination of net income on the accrual basis.

Materiality The concept that accounting should disclose those events that are relatively important to the practice or for understanding its statements.

Mixed cost A cost that has both fixed and variable cost attributes.

Modified accrual basis of accounting The basis of accounting under which depreciation is recognized on depreciable assets following accrual methods but some other expenses and/or revenues are recognized on a cash basis.

Net income The balance remaining to the owners of a practice after deducting from the gross revenue, for a given period, all operating expenses and income deductions during the same period.

Net lease Lease requiring payment, in addition to a fixed rental, of the expenses of the property leased, such as insurance, maintenance, taxes, and other similar obligations. The terms, net net, net net net, triple net are also used.

Net present value The present value of all future inflows, reduced at the appropriate discount rate, *minus* the present value of the cost (or costs) of the investment.

Nonoperating income Cash inflows from sources other than practice operations, for example parking-lot users' fees and building space rentals.

Operating cycle The period from the time resources are invested in performing a service until the time cash is recovered from the client.

Operating expenses The costs incurred in the process of providing services to patients, excluding costs pertaining to nonoperating activities such as general investments, endowments, etc.

Operational planning Process of predicting the needs for new personnel, facilities, and supplies; and when they should be budgeted.

Opportunity cost The benefit that would have been obtained from an alternative investment if that alternative had been chosen.

Organization costs The costs incurred in planning, organizing, and establishing a corporation (example of an intangible asset). The amounts are usually capitalized and written off over 60 months, the minimum period under U.S. tax law.

Overdraft The amount by which checks, drafts, or other demands for payment on a bank exceed the amount of the credit against which they are drawn.

Overhead Those elements of cost necessary in the performance of a service that do not become an integral part of the service, for example, rent, heat, electricity, management, and other similar costs. (See indirect expenses.)

Overtime Additional wages paid to employees of the practice for work performed in addition to the normal work period for which the employee is compensated.

Partnership Two or more veterinarians practicing under a contractual agreement as an unincorporated business.

Payback The length of time required for the net revenues generated by the investment to return the cost of the investment.

Payback period A capital budgeting technique that measures the length of time necessary to recover the initial investment in a project. Because discounted cash flow analysis is usually ignored in determining the payback period, it is a less desirable long-range decision technique than adjusted rate of return or net present value.

Pension plan Provisions of an employer's contract with employees for paying retirement annuities or other benefits.

Performance budget A budget prepared at the end of an accounting period for control purposes showing what revenues and costs should have been for the actual level of operations.

Periodic inventory A method of determining the ending inventory by taking a physical count of the material or supplies on hand at the end of the accounting period. For interim periods an estimate of inventory rather than actual count is often used.

Perpetual inventory A stock control system whereby the inventory of units of property at any date may be obtained directly from the records without resorting to an actual physical count. A record is maintained for each item or group of items to be inventoried and is so divided as to provide a running record of goods ordered, received, withdrawn, and the balance on hand in units and frequently also in value.

Petty cash A sum of money set aside for the purpose of paying small obligations for which the issuance of formal vouchers and checks would be too expensive and time-consuming. The petty cash fund should be reimbursed at the end of the monthly accounting period and when the fund is low. The expense (or other account) is recorded at the time of reimbursement. (See imprest fund.)

Planning The selection or identification of the long-range goals, priorities, and objectives of the organization and the formulation of various courses of action in terms of needs and relative costs or benefits to be followed in working toward achieving these goals, priorities, and objectives.

Posting The act of transferring to an account in a ledger the detailed or summarized data contained in the cash receipts book, check register, journal voucher, or similar books or documents of original entry.

Prepaid expenses Under accrual accounting, payment for goods or services that will provide benefits to the practice within the next operating cycle, e.g., insurance prepayments.

Present value (PV) The value today of a payment (or stream of payments) received at a future time, reduced by the appropriate discount rate.

Prime rate The interest rate for loans charged by commercial banks to their most preferred risks.

Professional corporation (PC) A legal entity created and operated under authority of the state through the articles of incorporation. A professional corporation requires shareholders to be licensed in the same profession (veterinary medicine, dentistry, architecture, etc).

Profit The excess of revenues over expenses for a period of time. (See income and net income.)

Profit center A responsibility center that performs a service to patients and to which revenues, as well as costs, can be traced.

Pro-forma statements Projections of future financial activities or positions based on past performance; in the case of new businesses, estimates of future financial activity.

Purchase option The right granted to the lessee by the lessor to purchase the leased assets at a previously agreed-upon or negotiated price.

Qualified opinion Auditor's report containing a statement that the auditor was unable to complete a satisfactory examination of all he thinks relevant or that he has doubts about the financial impact of some item or its validity as reported in the financial statements.

Receipts The cash inflow (or positive cash flow) that occurs as the result of either 1) revenue from prepayments or fees-for-service (operating receipts) or 2) proceeds from external sources such as grants, donations, and loans (nonoperating receipts).

Record management The maintenance of records and files on patients. It includes file updating and record retention.

Refund An amount paid back or credit allowed because of an overcollection.

Relevant range The span of volume over which cost behavior (or management plans) can be expected to remain valid.

Renewal option The right that is granted a lessee at the end of the initial lease term to renew the lease at pre-agreed or negotiated rates.

Rent Payment for the use, rather than ownership, of an asset (lease).

Reorder point In materials management, a stockage level at which a new order should be placed. The time to order and receive the stock, as well as a safety margin, is considered in setting the stockage level. (See economic order quantity [EOQ])

Requisition A written request, usually from a department to the purchasing officer or to another department, for specified articles or services.

Residual value Value of a leased asset at the end of the basic lease term.

Resource A generic term used to describe any type of manpower, facility, equipment, supply, or service having a monetary value (or cost) and required by the practice in order to function.

Retained earnings In the equity section of the balance sheet, the accumulation year to year of any net income that a corporation has chosen not to pay out as dividends to shareholders.

Return on investment The monetary gain from money or resources invested.

Revenue The increase in assets through the provision of goods or services. On the cash basis it is measured as the cash collected from clients regardless of when service was performed. On the accrual basis it is measured as the value of services provided to patients.

Salary The total amount regularly paid or stipulated to be paid to an individual, before deductions, for personal services rendered while on the payroll of the practice.

Sale-leaseback A financing transaction where improved property is sold, usually to a financial institution, then leased back to the prior owner. If the transaction is in substance a loan, the asset and the loan will be recorded in the accounts with lease payments treated as principal and interest payments on the loan and depreciation recorded for the asset.

Self-insurance The assumption of the financial risk by an individual or organization rather than purchasing coverage from an insurance carrier.

Semivariable costs Costs containing both fixed and variable components.

Short-range decisions Decisions involving service mix, volume of services, pricing, and distribution of profit. These decisions are concerned with the optimum use of existing resources and usually the time value of money is not considered significant. Also called operating decisions.

Simple interest Interest calculated on average unpaid (loan or investment) principal balance over its full term.

Sinking fund A fund established solely to pay off the principal of a loan when it falls due. The fund is normally accumulated by periodic transfer of monies equivalent to the depreciation allowable on the asset for which the loan was established.

Sole proprietorship A single veterinarian owning an unincorporated practice that may or may not have other veterinarians as employees.

Solo practitioner A self-employed veterinarian who may or may not be incorporated but who practices by himself.

Source document The underlying form or document for an accounting entry; an original record.

Standard A precise measure of what should occur if performance is efficient; it may be for nonfinancial as well as financial measures.

Statement of assets and liabilities A cash-basis position statement that shows the assets (resources) and the liabilities (claims against resources) of an organization at a specific time.

Statement of changes in financial position A general purpose financial statement on the accrual basis that explains the changes in working capital (or cash) during an accounting period.

Statement of revenues collected and expenses A cash-basis operating statement that shows the amount of cash collected, cash expenses paid, and depreciation expense for a period.

Statement of financial position See balance sheet.

Straight-line depreciation Depreciation technique providing for equal write-down of asset cost each year of the depreciable life of asset.

Tangible property Assets with physical characteristics, including plant, property, and equipment.

Time value of money The difference between the value of a dollar today and its value at some future point in time if invested now.

Trade discount An allowance, usually varying in percentage with volume of transactions, made to those engaged in certain businesses and allowable irrespective of the time when the account is paid. The term should not be confused with cash discount.

Trial balance A list of the balances of the accounts in a ledger kept by double entry, with the debit and credit balances shown in separate columns. If the totals of the debit and credit columns are equal or their net balance agrees with a controlling account, the ledger from which the figures are taken is said to be in balance.

Turnover The number of times that assets, such as accounts receivable, are replaced during a period. Accounts receivable turnover, for example, is total billings on account for a period divided by average accounts receivable balance for the period.

Unit cost Total cost of a function, activity, or service divided by the number of times the function, activity, or service was provided.

Unsecured loan A loan granted without collateral or security; generally a small loan secured by the signature and good credit of the borrower.

Variable costs Costs that vary in total dollar amount in direct proportion changes in activity. The variable cost per unit of output is assumed to be constant over the relevant range of activity.

Variance The difference between actual results and planned results.

Vested benefits Pension plan benefits that are not contingent on the employee continuing to work for the employer.

Voucher A document that authorizes the payment of money and usually indicates the accounts to be charged.

Withholding The process of deducting from a salary an amount specified by law, regulation, contract, or employee request.

Working capital The excess of total current assets over total current liabilities.

Write-off method The recognition of an uncollectible account receivable as a loss as determined by the time the specific account receivable has been identified as uncollectible.

Appendix F

MEDICAL RECORD AND LOG FORMS

SINGLE ANIMAL RECORD

OWNER'S NAME ______________________________ CASE NO. __________

ADDRESS ______________________ TEL. ______________ REF. BY __________

SPECIES ______________ BREED ______________ NAME ______________

SEX ________ AGE ________ COLOR AND MARKINGS ______________________

DATE			DESCRIPTION	CHARGE		PAID		BALANCE	
MO.	DAY	YR.							

ANCOM® BUSINESS SYSTEMS 65-0012 1981 SYMATIC, INC., HINCKLEY, OHIO

reprinted with permission of Ancom Business Products 800/845-9010

DATE			DESCRIPTION	CHARGE		PAID		BALANCE	
MO.	DAY	YR.							

reprinted with permission of Ancom Business Products 800/845-9010

Sample Single Animal Record (front and back)

OUT OUT OUT OUT OUT OUT OUT

OWNER'S NAME			PATIENT NO.
ADDRESS	CITY	STATE	ZIP
		HOME PHONE	BUS. PHONE

NAME	BREED	SEX	BORN	COLOR

DATE →												
RABIES												
DHL / FDV												
FECAL EXAM												
HEARTWORM B. T.												
DENTAL HYG.												
ANNUAL PHYSICAL												
WEIGHT												
PARVO												

JAN.	0
FEB.	1
MAR.	2
APR.	3
MAY	4
JUN.	5
JUL.	6
AUG.	7
SEP.	8
OCT.	9
NOV.	
DEC.	

ABNORMALITIES AND IDIOSYNCRASIES	NO.	DATE	PROBLEM LIST
	1		
	2		
	3		
	4		
MEDICATION	5		
	6		
	7		
	8		
	9		
	10		
	11		
X-RAYS DIAGNOSIS	12		
	13		
	14		
	15		
	16		
	17		
DIET	18		
	19		
	20		

COUNTY ANIMAL HOSPITAL
NEW CITY, N. Y.

9 x 8 – .75
132
N 17109 A

Sample Medical Record (front)

OWNER'S NAME

NAME

Minimum Data Base (CBC, urinalysis, fecal)
SOAP (Subjective, Objective, Assessment, Plan-Diagnostic (Dx), Therapeutic (Rx), Client Ed (CE)).
DAMN IT (Degenerative, Anomalies, Autoimmune, Metabolic, Neoplasia, Inflammatory, Immune disorders, Trauma, Toxicity).

PHYSICAL EXAM | Temp. (T), Pulse (P), Resp. (R), Eye (Ey), Ear (Ea), Nose (No), Mucous Membranes (MM), Teeth (Te), Pharynx (Ph), Lymph Nodes (LN), Hydration (Hy), Upper Respiratory Tract (URT), Heart (H), Lungs (L), Abdomen (Ab), Genitalia (Ge), Musculo-Skeletal (MS), Skin (Sk), Nervous (Ne).

DATE	T	A	B		CODE	CHARGE

Sample Medical Record (back)

SINGLE ANIMAL RECORD

Owner____________________ Patient's Name ____________________

Address____________________ City/State ____________________ Zip __________

Phone: Home____________________ Business ____________________

Species ____________________ Breed ____________________

Color____________________ Sex __________ Birth Date ____________________

Individual Needs ________ ________ ________ ________

Diet ____________________
Coat Supplement ____________________
Flea ____________________
Vitamins ____________________
Shampoo ____________________

Physical Exam: **N** — normal **A** — abnormal **NE** — not examined

Date	/	/	/	/	/	/	/	/	/	/	/	/	/	/	/	/	/	/	/	/	/	/	/	/	/
General appearance & Temp																									
Integumentary																									
Eyes																									
Ears																									
Nose & Throat																									
Mucous membranes & Teeth																									
Musculoskeletal																									
Circulatory																									
Digestive																									
Respiratory																									
Genito-urinary																									
Anal sacs																									
Neural system																									
Lymph nodes																									
Weight																									

Date		Description	Vaccinations/Fecal
In	Out		

ANCOM BUSINESS SYSTEMS Form No. 65-8010

Sample Single Animal Record form

OWNER/PATIENT RECORD

ANCOM 8400

OWNER MS MISS MR MRS DR ____ PATIENT'S NAME ____

ADDRESS ____ CITY ____ ZIP ____

PHONE HOME ____ BUSINESS ____ BEST TIME TO CALL ____

SPECIES ____ COLOR ____ SEX ____ BIRTH DATE ____

BREED ____ IMMUNIZATION RECORD DHL ____ DHLP ____ MEASLES ____

WEIGHT ____ HEARTWORM ____ F D ____ FVR-CV ____ RABIES ____

HISTORY

PREVIOUS PROBLEMS ____

CURRENT PROBLEMS ____

SPECIAL PROBLEMS

DATE MO	DATE DAY	DATE YR	PROBLEM NUMBER	SOAP FORMAT	PROGRESS NOTES	FEE		PAID		BALANCE	

Sample Owner/Patient Record

FORM NO. 65-8410

PROGRESS NOTES

PAGE ______

OWNER'S NAME	PATIENT'S NAME	BREED	COLOR	SEX	BIRTH DATE

DATE			PROBLEM NUMBER	SOAP FORMAT	PROGRESS NOTES	FEE	PAID	BALANCE
MO.	DAY	YR.						

reprinted with permission of Ancom Business Products 800/845-9010

Sample Progress Notes form

AAHA®
AMERICAN ANIMAL HOSPITAL ASSOCIATION

S = Subjective (complaint/history)
O = Objective (exam)
A = Assessment (diagnosis, R/O)
P = Plan (action/C.E.)

PROGRESS NOTES

CANINE DENTAL

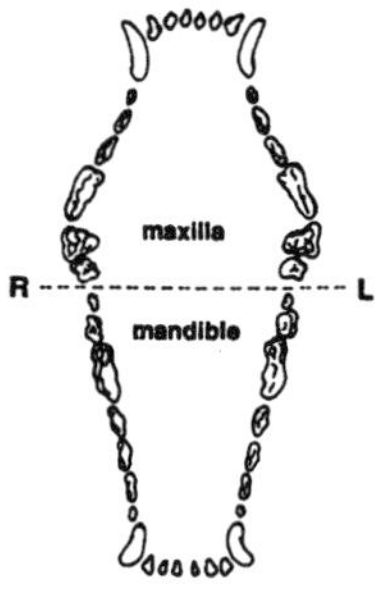

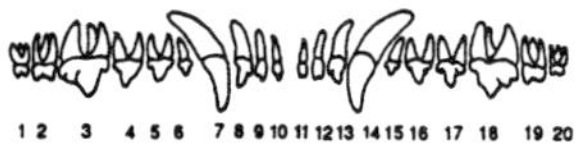

KEY: P = POCKETS
O = EXTRACTED TOOTH
X = MISSING TOOTH

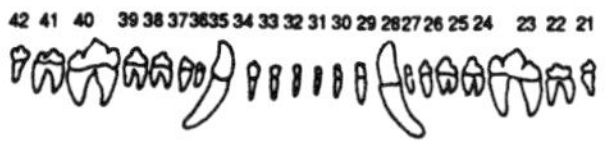

AAHA-PMST 2/95 - 50M

SURGICAL SUMMARY

NAME ______ DATE ______
Lab: Y N
PROCEDURE: ______ X-rays: Y N
Pre-Anesth: ______
Induction: ______ mask/tube
Anesth: ______ Time: ______
Monitor Sys: ______
Surgeon: ______ Asst: ______
Surgical Observation:

Fluids: ______
CLOSURE:
Musc. ______
Periton. ______
SubQ ______
Skin ______

AAHA-PMSS 2/93 50M

FELINE DENTAL

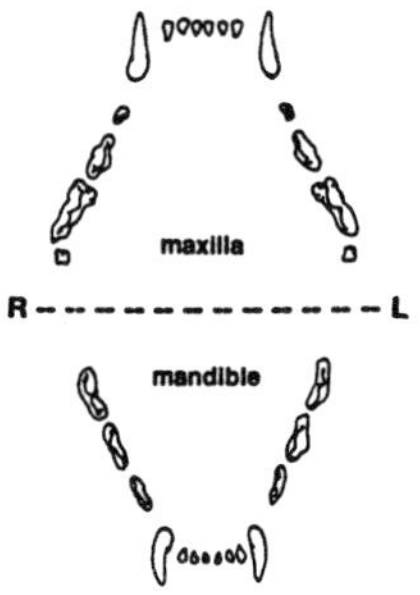

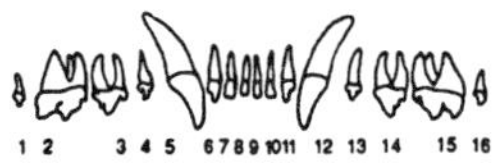

KEY: P = POCKETS
O = EXTRACTED TOOTH
X = MISSING TOOTH

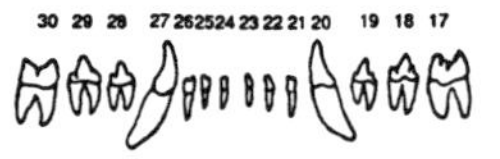

AAHA-PMST 2/95 - 50M

AUTHORIZATION TO PERFORM EUTHANASIA

I, the undersigned, am the owner/duly authorized agent for the owner of the animal described hereon. I verify that said pet has not bitten any person or animal during the last fourteen (14) days and to the best of my knowledge has not been exposed to rabies. I hereby consent to and order euthanasia (humane death) to be performed on this animal forever releasing said doctor and his agent from any and all liability for performing said euthanasia.

It is my desire to provide for my pet decent and humane after-death care, complying with all legal requirements of the area. I authorize the attending veterinarian to now dispose of the remains in accordance with hospital policy, releasing the hospital, doctor, and agents from any and all liability for performing said after-death care, with the following stipulations included:

____ return remains for personal disposition
____ communal burial or group disposal (legal definitions)
____ cremation (____communal____private____returned ashes)
____ postmortem evaluation prior to the above disposition.

Signature ______ Date ______

AAHA-PMEU 6/90-25M

Sample Progress Notes Stickers (page 1 of 2)

AAHA® AMERICAN ANIMAL HOSPITAL ASSOCIATION

S = Subjective (complaint/history)
O = Objective (exam)
A = Assessment (diagnosis, R/O)
P = Plan (action/C.E.)

PROGRESS NOTES

Physical Exam Checklist

1) GENERAL APPEARANCE	2) ORAL CAVITY	3) TEETH	4) EYES
☐ NRM ☐ ABN ☐ NE	☐ NRM ☐ ABN ☐ NE	☐ NRM ☐ ABN ☐ NE	☐ NRM ☐ ABN ☐ NE
5) EARS	6) HEART	7) RESPIRATORY	8) ABDOMEN
☐ NRM ☐ ABN ☐ NE	☐ NRM ☐ ABN ☐ NE	☐ NRM ☐ ABN ☐ NE	☐ NRM ☐ ABN ☐ NE
9) MUSCULOSKELETAL	10) LYMPH NODES	11) GENITOURINARY	12) INTEGUMENTARY
☐ NRM ☐ ABN ☐ NE	☐ NRM ☐ ABN ☐ NE	☐ NRM ☐ ABN ☐ NE	☐ NRM ☐ ABN ☐ NE

T______ **P**______ **R**______ **Wt.**______ **DIET**______

INDOOR ◄──► OUTDOOR OTHER

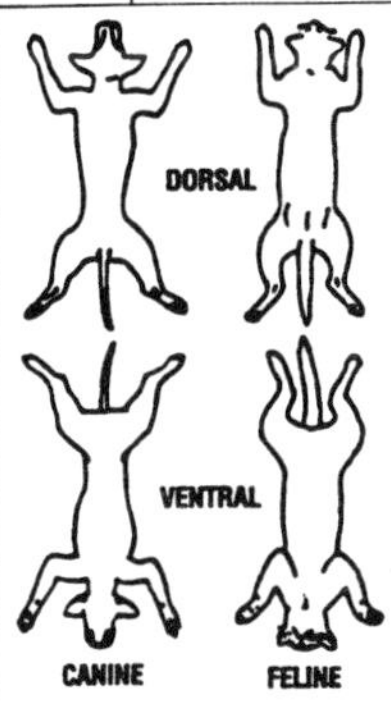

DERMATOLOGY

LESIONS (circle): Photos ☐

Macules Papules Pustules Vesicles
Crusts Excoriations Ulcers Scales
Pruritis Wheals Nodules Tumors ( )
Lichenification Hyperpigmentation
Erythema Alopecia Hyperkeratosis

Fleas Lice Sarcoptes Demodex Ticks

Fungi: Woods _____ KOH _____ Culture _____

Bacteriology: __________

Direct Smear: __________

Biopsy: __________

Lab: Out __________ In __________

AAHA-PMSD 12/93-100M

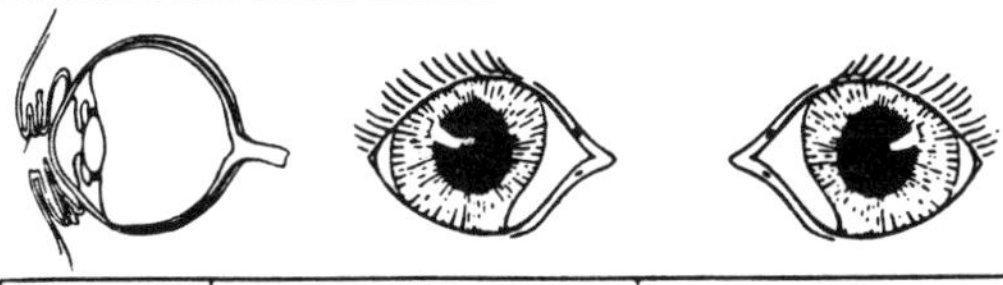

AAHA-PMSD 12/93-100M

OPHTHALMOLOGY	RIGHT	LEFT
EYE POSITION		
LIDS		
SCLERA		
CONJUNCTIVA		
TEARS		
LENS		
IRIS		
PUPIL		
RETINA		

Sample Progress Notes Stickers (page 2 of 2)

DATE ______________ **MASTER PROBLEM LIST** PAGE ______

OWNER'S NAME	PATIENT'S NAME	BREED	COLOR	SEX	BIRTH DATE

PROBLEM NUMBER	MAJOR PROBLEM (LASTING EFFECT)	DATE NOTICED	⟶ ⟵	DATE RESOLVED
1				
2				
3				
4				
5				
6				
7				
8				
9				
10				
11				
12				
13				
14				
15				

MINOR PROBLEM LIST

PROBLEM NO.	PROBLEM TEMPORARY, ACUTE, OR SELF-LIMITING	DATES OF OCCURRENCE				
		1	2	3	4	5
A						
B						
C						
D						
E						
F						
G						
H						
I						
J						
K						
L						
M						
N						
O						

reprinted with permission of Ancom Business Products 800/845-9010

Sample Medical Record form (front)

MEDICATION LIST

MEDICATION	DATE BEGUN	RESPONSE	DATE BEGUN	RESPONSE	DATE BEGUN	RESPONSE

ANCOM BUSINESS SYSTEMS FORM NO. 65-8450

Sample Medical Record form (back)

FORM NO. 65-8410

PROGRESS NOTES

PAGE ______

OWNER'S NAME	PATIENT'S NAME	BREED	COLOR	SEX	BIRTH DATE

DATE			PROBLEM NUMBER	SOAP FORMAT	PROGRESS NOTES	FEE		PAID		BALANCE	
MO	DAY	YR									

Sample Progress Notes form

DATE ____________

DERMATOLOGICAL EXAMINATION

ANCOM BUSINESS SYSTEMS FORM NO. 65-8490

OWNER'S NAME	PATIENT'S NAME	BREED	COLOR	SEX	BIRTH DATE

HAIR COAT LENGTH ____ CONDITION ____ ALOPECIA ____

SKIN PRURITIS ____ MACULES ____ HYPERPIGMENTATION ____ TUMORS ____
ERYTHEMIA ____ PAPULES ____ HYPERKERATOSIS ____ CYSTS ____
EXCORIATION ____ PUSTULES ____ LICHENIFICATION ____ OTHER LESIONS ____
ABRASIONS ____ WHEELS ____ SCALES ____

ECTOPARASITES FLEAS TICKS LICE SCABIES DEMODEX SCRAPING LOCATION ____

FUNGI WOOD'S LIGHT ____ KOH ____ CULTURE ____ METH. BLUE ____

SYSTEMIC THYROID PROFILE ____ IMMUNE PROFILE ____

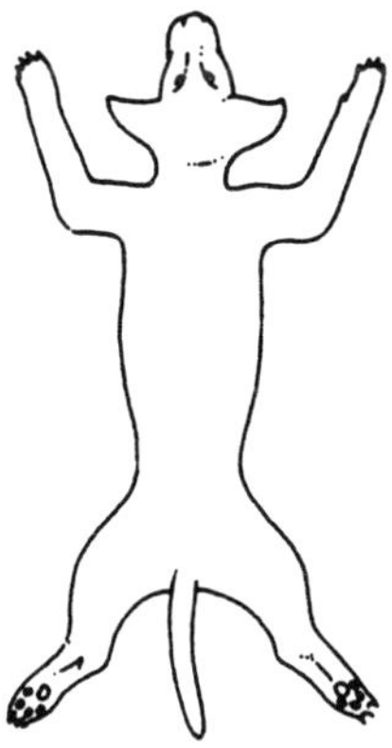

DORSAL

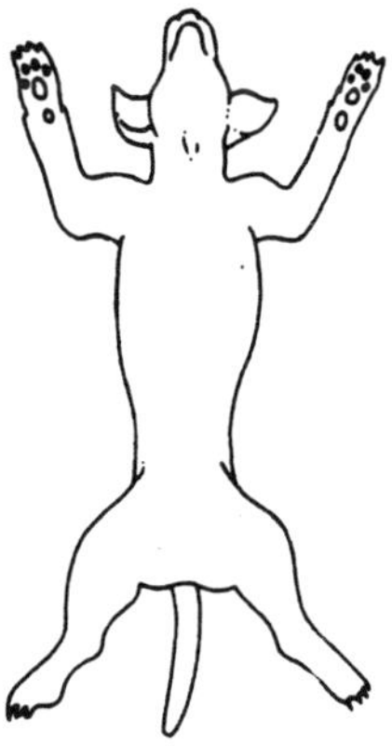

VENTRAL

COMMENTS:

reprinted with permission of Ancom Business Products 800/845-9010

Sample Dermatological Examination form

DATE ______ **RADIOGRAPHIC EVALUATION** NUMBER ______

OWNER'S NAME	PATIENT'S NAME	BREED	COLOR	SEX	BIRTH DATE

MACHINE SETTING CM ______ KV ______ MAS ______ MA ______ SEC ______

TECHNIQUE POSITION

INTERPRETATION

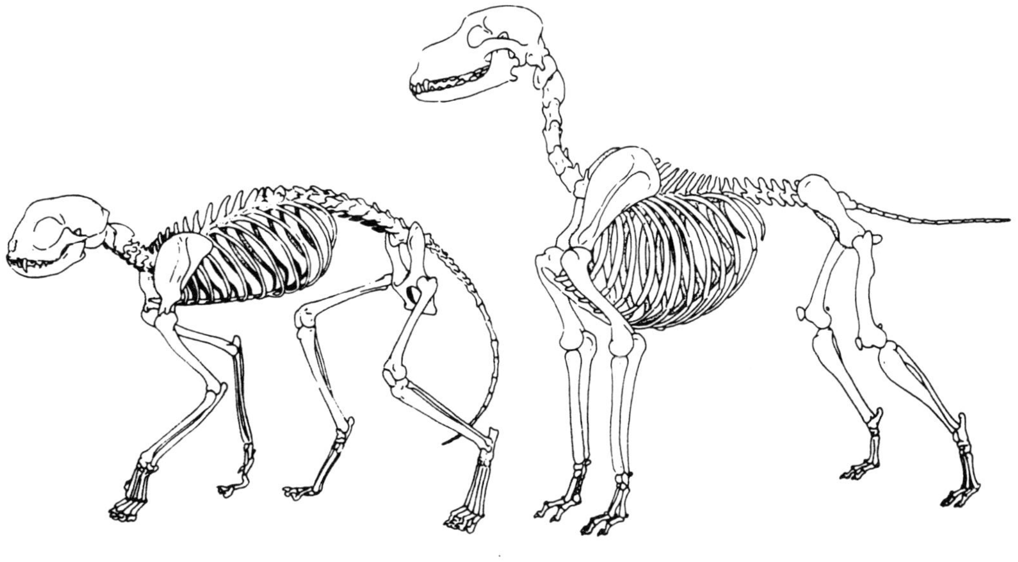

ANCOM BUSINESS SYSTEMS FORM NO 65-8500

reprinted with permission of Ancom Business Products 800/845-9010

Sample Radiographic Evaluation form

DATE ____________

OPHTHALMOLOGICAL EXAMINATION

OWNER'S NAME	PATIENT'S NAME	BREED	COLOR	SEX	BIRTH DATE

	LEFT	RIGHT
LIDS	N A UPPER ☐ ☐ LOWER ☐ ☐ THIRD ☐ ☐	N A ☐ ☐ ☐ ☐ ☐ ☐
SCLERA	NORMAL ☐ INJECTED ☐ ICTERIC ☐	NORMAL ☐ INJECTED ☐ ICTERIC ☐
CONJUNCTIVA	N A ☐ ☐	N A ☐ ☐
CORNEA	◯	◯
LENS	☐ NORMAL ☐ CATARACT ☐ LENTICULAR SCLEROSIS	☐ NORMAL ☐ CATARACT ☐ LENTICULAR SCLEROSIS
IRIS	N A ☐ ☐	N A ☐ ☐
PUPIL	EQUAL UNEQUAL LIGHT RESPONSE	EQUAL UNEQUAL LIGHT RESPONSE
RETINA	VESSELS OPTIC DISK	VESSELS OPTIC DISK
TEAR PRODUCTION	N A ☐ ☐	N A ☐ ☐
EYE POSITION	☐ NORMAL ☐ CROSSED ☐ DIVERGENT	☐ NORMAL ☐ CROSSED ☐ DIVERGENT

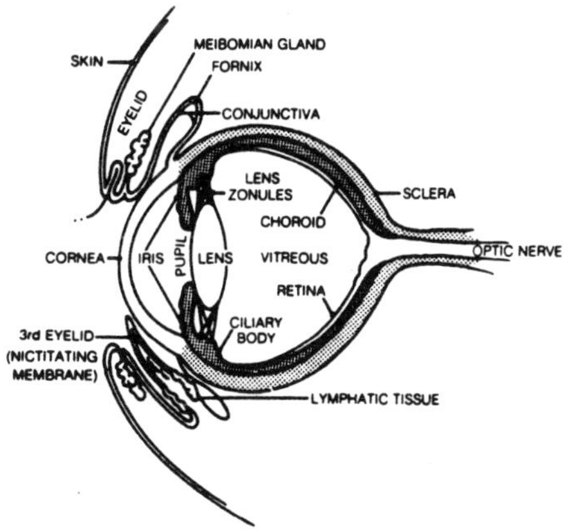

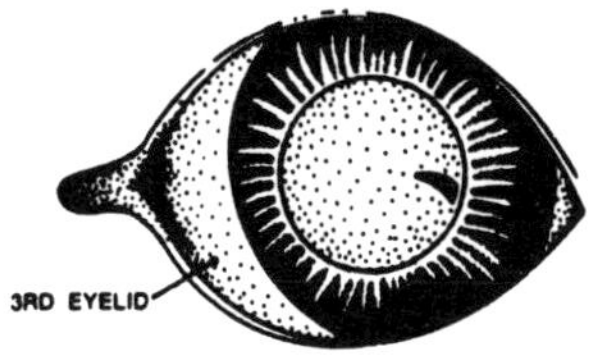

ANCOM BUSINESS SYSTEMS

FORM NO. 65-8510

Sample Ophthalmological Examination form

DATE ____________

CARDIO-VASCULAR EVALUATION

OWNER'S NAME	PATIENT'S NAME	BREED	COLOR	SEX	BIRTH DATE

PALPATION

HEART N ☐ A ☐ DESCRIBE ____________

PULSE ☐ NORMAL ☐ WEAK ☐ STRONG ☐ ARRHYTHMIA FEMORAL ____ MIN. JUGULAR VENOUS ____________

AUSCULTATION

HEART SOUNDS	MURMUR	DURATION	PITCH	LOUDNESS	AREA	
NORMAL ☐	SYSTOLIC ☐	EARLY ☐	HIGH ☐	SOFT ☐	PULMONIC ☐	MITRIAL ☐
ABNORMAL ☐	DIASTOLIC ☐	LATE ☐	LOW ☐	MEDIUM ☐	AORTIC ☐	TRICUSPID ☐
MURMUR ☐	CONTINUOUS ☐		MIXED ☐	LOUD ☐		

LUNG CONDITION
☐ DRY
☐ MOIST
☐ PULMONARY EDEMA

COUGH
☐ A.M. ☐ PRODUCTIVE
☐ P.M. ☐ NON-PRODUCTIVE
☐ NOCTURNAL

E.C.G.

HEART RATE ____________ RHYTHM ____________

P ________ P-R ________ QRS ________ QT ________ ST-T ________

AXIS ____________

OTHER:

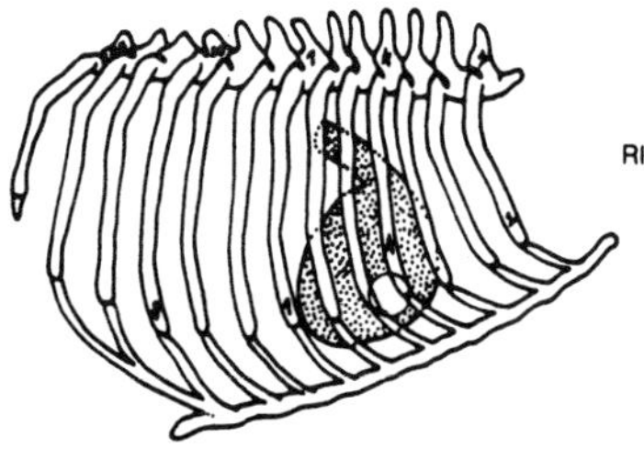

RIGHT

LEFT

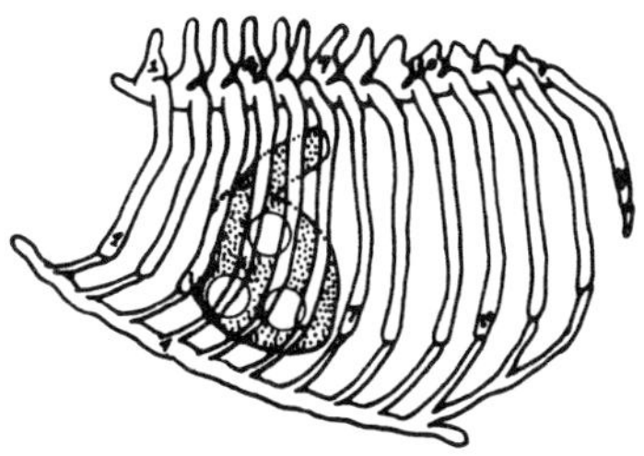

COMMENTS:

ANCOM BUSINESS SYSTEMS

FORM NO. 65-852C

reprinted with permission of Ancom Business Products 800/845-9010

Sample Cardiovascular Evaluation form

DATE ____________

NEUROLOGICAL EXAMINATION

OWNER'S NAME	PATIENT'S NAME	BREED	COLOR	SEX	BIRTH DATE

GENERAL OBSERVATIONS	N	A
MENTAL STATUS	☐	☐
DISPOSITION	☐	☐
GAIT AND POSTURE	☐	☐

	NO	YES
HEAD TRAUMA	☐	☐

SEIZURES FREQUENCY ____________

DURATION ________ AURA________ SEIZURE________ POSTICTAL

LOSS OF CONSCIOUSNESS NO ☐ YES ☐ ____________

MUSCLE TONE N ☐ A ☐ ____________

DISK SYNDROME ☐ SPINAL ☐ CERVICAL

SPINAL REFLEXES				
PATELLAR		L		R
BICEPS		L		R
TRICEPS		L		R
PERINEAL				
FLEXOR	LF	LR	RF	RR
CROSSED EXTENSOR				
PAIN PERCEPTION				

POSTURAL REACTIONS				
HOPPING	LF	RF	LR	RR
EXTENSOR POSTURAL THRUST			LR	RR
HEMI-STANDS			L	R
HEMI-WALKS			L	R
PROPRIOCEPTIVE POSITIONING	LF	RF	LR	RR
PLACING: OPTIC	LF	RF	LR	RR
TACTILE	LF	RF	LR	RR
WHEELBARROWING				
TONIC NECK AND EYE				

CRANIAL NERVES		
1. OLFACTORY		1. ANOSMIA
2. OPTIC		2. BLINDNESS, MYDRIASIS if Bil.
3. OCULOMOTOR		3. MYDRIASIS, PTOSIS, EYE ROTATION
4. TROCHLEAR		4. EYE UNABLE TO MOVE VENTROLATERALLY
5. TRIGEMINAL		5. MOTOR-WEAKNESS CLOSING MOUTH SENSORY—NO SENSATION, FACE & EYE
6. ABDUCENS		6. EYE FAILS TO MOVE LATERALLY
7. FACIAL		7. PARALYSIS: FACE, LIPS, EYELIDS, EARS
8. ACOUSTIC		8. DEAFNESS, HEAD TILT, CIRCLING
9. GLOSSOPHARYNGEAL		9. DIFFICULTY EATING
10. VAGUS		10. SAGGING SOFT PALATE
11. SPINAL ACCESSORY		11. DEVIATION OF HEAD TO SIDE
12. HYPOGLOSSAL		12. TONGUE PROTRUDES ON AFFECTED SIDE

COMMENTS:

ANCOM BUSINESS SYSTEMS

FORM NO. 65-8580

Sample Neurological Examination form

AAHA
AMERICAN ANIMAL HOSPITAL ASSOCIATION

PRESURGICAL CARE

Patient____________________________ Date of Sugery ___/___/___ Time _________

Please read and follow the steps outlined to prepare your pet for surgery. This information is provided with your pet's safety in mind.

No food after _________ am/pm the day of/before surgery.
No water or other liquids after _________ am/pm the day of/before surgery.
Drop off your pet by ____________ am/pm on the day of surgery.
You may call after ____________ am/pm to obtain your pet's condition and tentative release time.
____Vaccinations are current until ______________.
____ We have no record of your pet's vaccination (please bring proof).

HOSPITAL/SURGICAL INFORMATION

- Preparation — The skin surrounding the surgical area will be clipped and scrubbed with an antiseptic. Equipment used will be sterilized, and surgery personnel will antiseptically scrub and wear gloves, masks, gowns and caps during the operation.
- Anesthesia — Local or general anesthesia may be used. Somc risk is involved, depending upon the general condition of your pet, age, etc. Surgery may occur as scheduled or be delayed, depending upon the determination after presurgical examination.
- Heart/Respiration — Monitoring of these functions will occur during the operation.

POSTSURGICAL CARE

Both staff and doctor will check your pet routinely during the hospital stay, and again just prior to discharge. We will meet with you before taking your pet home, and give you postsurgical information. If you wish to discuss this only with the doctor, please make advance arrangements.

#235 7/91

Sample Presurgical Care form

American Animal Hospital Association

1 2 3 4 5 6 7 8 9 10 11 12 13 **Patient Data**

Owner's Name ______________________ Pet's Name ______________

Address ______________________ City ______________

State/Prov ______________________ Zip/PC ______________

Phone: (H) ____________ (B) ____________ Breed ____________

Color ____________ Born ____________ Sex ____________

Idiosyncrasis ______________________________________

Health Maintenance	Date ☛											
Rabies												
Distemper/Respir Multivalent Vac												
FIP/Corona Vac												
FeLV/Parvo Vac												
FTLV/Bordetella Vac												
Annual Physical												
Heartworm Test/FeLV Test												
Fecal Exam												
Weight												
Dental Hygiene												
Diet												
Surgery Date												
X-ray Date												

ALERT DATA:

Date	#	Problem List	Resolved	Date	Medications

Sample Patient Data form

AAHA® AMERICAN ANIMAL HOSPITAL ASSOCIATION

S = Subjective (complaint/history)
O = Objective (exam)
A = Assessment (diagnosis, R/O)
P = Plan (action/C.E.)

PROGRESS NOTES

DATE	SOAP	

Sample Progress Notes form

AVIAN MINIMUM DEFINED DATA BASE

Date______Client#________

Owner________________Species____________Name____________

Sex____Age_____Source__________Obtained______Leg Band#______

Diet______seed%_____veg%_____other%,supplements______________

Other birds__________Cage condition&cups G/B/NA____________

Psittacosis discussed YN___Permission to test Y,N, WC ____________

History____

____

____

PHYSICAL EXAM Weight__________Gms.

Gen. Appear. N/Abn_______ N Thin Fat__

____

Integument N/Abn_______mites,tumor,beak,plumage-bright,dull,picking

____

Musc/Skel N/Abn_______Muscle mass,Perching,Lame,Wings

____

Respiratory N/Abn_______Nasal disch,Dyspnea,Lung/Airsac,Choana-wet/dry______

____

Cardiovasc N/Abn_______Anemia______________________

Digestive N/Abn._______Oral cavity,Regurg,Abd.palp,Feces______________

____

Eyes N/Abn_______Conjunctivitis,Ulcers______________

Urogenital N/Abn_______Urates,Egg bound______________

Neural N/Abn_______Seizures,Tremors______________

RADIOGRAPHIC RESULTS

____

____

LAB DATA REQUESTED-------Interpretation

CBC____Profile_________

Culture (bact./fung)_____

Gram Stain__________

Fecal (float/Trichrome)__

Psittacosis titer_________

PROBLEM LIST **BEGINNING THERAPY**

____

____

____

Sample Avian Medical Record form

AAHA® AMERICAN ANIMAL HOSPITAL ASSOCIATION

WT=Weight KV=Kilovolts SEC=Seconds
CM=Centimeters MA=Milliamps QNTY=Quantity

RADIOLOGY (IMAGING) LOG

DATE	IMAGE	PATIENT IDENTIFICATION	BREED	SEX	AGE	WT	VIEW	CM	KV	MA	SEC	QNTY / DIAGNOSIS / COMMENTS

 AMERICAN ANIMAL HOSPITAL ASSOCIATION 7/94

Sample Radiology (Imaging) Log form

AAHA® AMERICAN ANIMAL HOSPITAL ASSOCIATION

* Presurgical assessment

A. Minimal Risk
B. Slight risk
C. Moderate risk
D. High risk
E. Grave risk

SURGERY / ANESTHESIA LOG

DATE	PATIENT ID	* RISK	PREANES.	ANESTHESIA	PROCEDURE	ANES./SX. LENGTH	VOLUME DRAWN/USED	DR.	TECH

Sample Surgery/Anesthesia Log form

INTERNAL LABORATORY LOG
LABORATORY PURCHASE AND QUALITY CONTROL RECORD

PURCHASE DATE	REAGENT OR EQUIPMENT	LOT NO. OR SERIAL NO.	REAGENT QUALITY CONTROL										EQUIPMENT MAINTENANCE
			Date	Result	Date	Result	Date	Result	Date	Result	Date	Result	

Sample Internal Laboratory Log form (page 1 of 2)

SUMMARY	PCV	Hb	RBC	MCV	MCH	MCHC	PLAT	WBC	JUV	STAB	SEG	LYM	MONO	EOS	BASO	FILARIA	CLOT	OTHER
Month	U. COLOR	U. pH	U. PROT	U. GLU.	U. KET	OCC	U. BIL	UROB	S. GRAV	U. SED.				OTHER				
Year	CA	PHOS	GLU.	BUN	U.A.	CHOL	T. PROT	ALB.	BIL	A.P.	CREAT	OT/PT	AMYLASE	OTHER				
SUMMARY	PCV	Hb	RBC	MCV	MCH	MCHC	PLAT	WBC	JUV	STAB	SEG	LYM	MONO	EOS	BASO	FILARIA	CLOT	OTHER
Month	U. COLOR	U. pH	U. PROT	U. GLU.	U. KET	OCC	U. BIL	UROB	S. GRAV	U. SED.				OTHER				
Year	CA	PHOS	GLU.	BUN	U.A.	CHOL	T. PROT	ALB.	BIL	A.P.	CREAT	OT/PT	AMYLASE	OTHER				
SUMMARY	PCV	Hb	RBC	MCV	MCH	MCHC	PLAT	WBC	JUV	STAB	SEG	LYM	MONO	EOS	BASO	FILARIA	CLOT	OTHER
Month	U. COLOR	U. pH	U. PROT	U. GLU.	U. KET	OCC	U. BIL	UROB	S. GRAV	U. SED.				OTHER				
Year	CA	PHOS	GLU.	BUN	U.A.	CHOL	T. PROT	ALB.	BIL	A.P.	CREAT	OT/PT	AMYLASE	OTHER				
SUMMARY	PCV	Hb	RBC	MCV	MCH	MCHC	PLAT	WBC	JUV	STAB	SEG	LYM	MONO	EOS	BASO	FILARIA	CLOT	OTHER
Month	U. COLOR	U. pH	U. PROT	U. GLU.	U. KET	OCC	U. BIL	UROB	S. GRAV	U. SED.				OTHER				
Year	CA	PHOS	GLU.	BUN	U.A.	CHOL	T. PROT	ALB.	BIL	A.P.	CREAT	OT/PT	AMYLASE	OTHER				
SUMMARY	PCV	Hb	RBC	MCV	MCH	MCHC	PLAT	WBC	JUV	STAB	SEG	LYM	MONO	EOS	BASO	FILARIA	CLOT	OTHER
Month	U. COLOR	U. pH	U. PROT	U. GLU.	U. KET	OCC	U. BIL	UROB	S. GRAV	U. SED.				OTHER				
Year	CA	PHOS	GLU.	BUN	U.A.	CHOL	T. PROT	ALB.	BIL	A.P.	CREAT	OT/PT	AMYLASE	OTHER				
SUMMARY	PCV	Hb	RBC	MCV	MCH	MCHC	PLAT	WBC	JUV	STAB	SEG	LYM	MONO	EOS	BASO	FILARIA	CLOT	OTHER
Month	U. COLOR	U. pH	U. PROT	U. GLU.	U. KET	OCC	U. BIL	UROB	S. GRAV	U. SED.				OTHER				
Year	CA	PHOS	GLU.	BUN	U.A.	CHOL	T. PROT	ALB.	BIL	A.P.	CREAT	OT/PT	AMYLASE	OTHER				
SIX MONTH COMPOSITE	PCV	Hb	RBC	MCV	MCH	MCHC	PLAT	WBC	JUV	STAB	SEG	LYM	MONO	EOS	BASO	FILARIA	CLOT	OTHER
FROM / TO	U. COLOR	U. pH	U. PROT	U. GLU.	U. KET	OCC	U. BIL	UROB	S. GRAV	U. SED.				OTHER				
	CA	PHOS	GLU.	BUN	U.A.	CHOL	T. PROT	ALB.	BIL	A.P.	CREAT	OT/PT	AMYLASE	OTHER				

Sample Internal Laboratory Log form (page 2 of 2)

AAHA
AMERICAN ANIMAL HOSPITAL ASSOCIATION

EXTERNAL LABORATORY RECORD

DATE COLLECTED	CLIENT	PATIENT	TESTS REQUIRED	LAB ID	RESULTS (DATE)

Sample External Laboratory Record form

AMERICAN ANIMAL HOSPITAL ASSOCIATION

NECROPSY RECORD AND LOG

The potential value of the necropsy today is indisputable. It is of great importance in the teaching of medicine. It permits clinicians to test their acumen in the diagnosis of anatomic lesions, often at a cost of their pride, but with great gain in their wisdom. It instructs surgeons in the end results of their work. In other words, it is invaluable to the profession. It most benefits the clinician or surgeon who was attending the animal prior to death.

The necopsy record is intended to be used as the procedural guide to a complete well-documented necropsy. It represents a permanent record of objective, primarily morphological findings with little interpretation. Organs and leasions are described by (1) location and relationship to other organs and structures, (2) size, (3) weight, (4) shape, (5) color, (6) consistency, (7) odor, and (8) other special features, such as texture of cut surfaces. Descriptions should be brief yet complete. There should be no interpretations and no descriptions of the mechanics of dissection. Sizes should be stated in centimeters, and comparisons with fruits and other objects should be highly scientific and legally protective.

Write "N" for normal appearing organs, briefly describe the abnormal and leave blank if not examined. The record does not need to be typed but must be legibly written and signed if more than one person performs necropsies.

The necropsy log is to be used as an index of the necropsies performed, listing the major problems found or the causes of death. The complete record is filed in a notebook in chronological order.

References

1. Ludwig, J.: Current Methods of Autopsy Practice, Philadelphia, W.B. Saunders Co., 1972, pp. 263-265.
2. Starr, I.: Potential values of the autopsy today. ***JAMA 160***: 1144-1145, 1956.
3. Van Kruiningen, H.J.: Veterinary Autopsy Procedure, In: The Veterinary Clinics of North America, R.W. Kirk, editor, Philadelphia, W.B. Saunders Co., 1971, Vol 1, pp. 163-189.

Sample Introduction to Necropsy Log

NECROPSY LOG

Date	Case No.	Owner	Animal	Breed	Sex	Age	Necropsy Summary

Sample Necropsy Log form (page 1 of 2)

NECROPSY RECORD

Date	Case No.	Owner	Animal	Breed	Sex	Age	Weight	Markings
History Summary								
Date, Time, Manner of Death								
Necropsy Summary								

GROSS NECROPSY EXAMINATION		LABORATORY EXAMINATION
General Appearance	Urogenital System	Laboratory Data
Skin	Liver, Pancreas	Histopathology
Thoracic Cavity	Spleen, Lymph Nodes	Microbiology
Nasal Passages, Trachea, Bronchi	Endocrine System	Disposition of Carcass
Lungs	Central Nervous System	Owner Notification
Cardiovascular System	Sensory Organs	General Impressions (Subjective Evaluation)
Abdominal Cavity	Muscular System	
Mouth, Esophagus, Stomach	Skeletal System	
Small Intestine	Mammary Glands	
Large Intestine, Colon	Other	Signature

American Animal Hospital Association, 1978

Sample Necropsy Log form (page 2 of 2)

Appendix G

INVENTORY CONTROL CARD

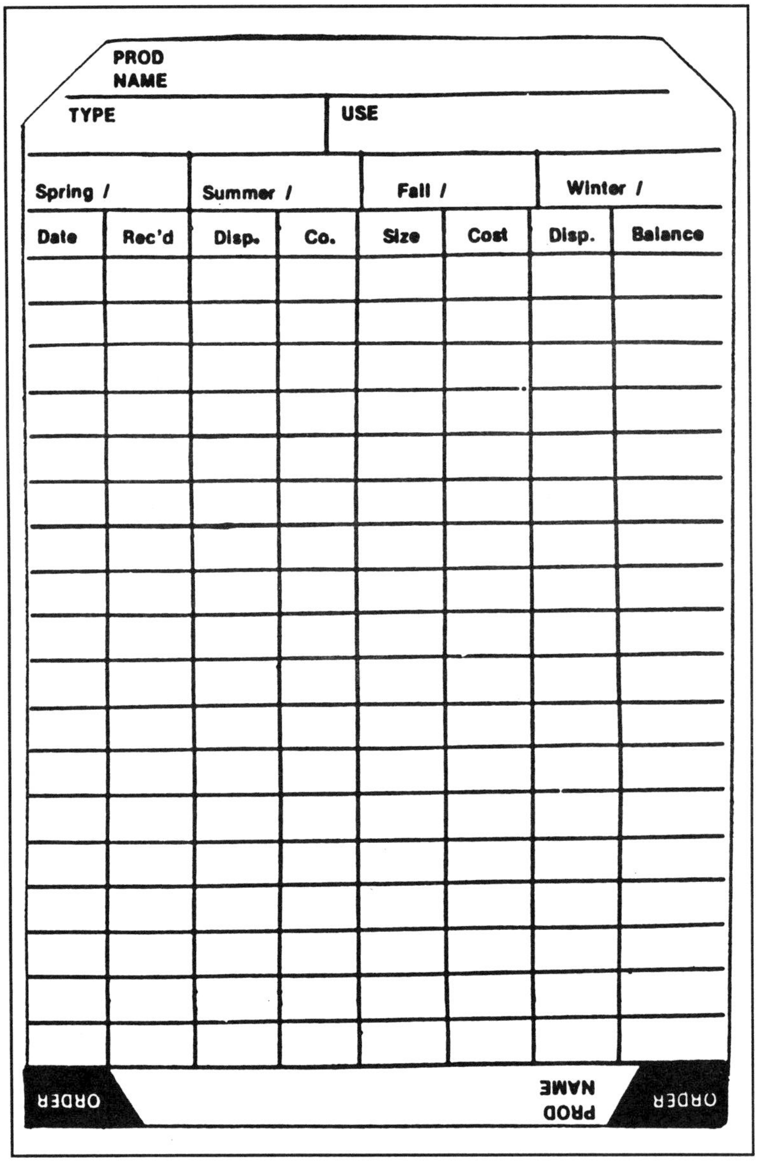

Sample Inventory Control card

Turn card upside-down when reorder needed.

Appendix H

THE HUMAN-COMPANION ANIMAL BOND RESOURCES

Books

Animals and People Sharing the World, Andrew N. Rowan, University Press of New England for Tufts University, 1988

Between Pets and People, Alan Beck and Aaron Katcher, G.P. Putnam's Sons, 1983

Good-Bye My Friend - Grieving the Death of a Pet, Mary & Herb Montgomery, Available through the American Animal Hospital Association, Montgomery Press, 1991

I'll Always Love You - Children's Pet Loss Book, Hans Wilhelm, Crown Publishers, Inc., New York, NY, 1985

New Perspectives of Our Lives with Companion Animals, Aaron Katcher and Alan Beck, University of Pennsylvania Press, 1983

On Death and Dying, Elizabeth Kubler-Ross, Macmillan Publishing, 1969

Pet Loss - A Thoughtful Guide for Adults and Children, Herbert Neiberg, Harper and Row, 1982

Problems in Veterinary Medicine - "Animal Illness and Human Emotion," Susan Phillips Cohen, MSW, and Carole E. Fudin, PhD, J.B. Lippincott, 1991

The Tenth Good Thing About Barney - Children's Pet Loss Book, Judith Viorst, Aladdin Books, Macmillan Publishing Co., 1988

The Veterinary Clinics of North America - "The Human-Companion Animal Bond," Vol 15, No 2, March 1985, Jamie Quackenbush and Victoria Voith, W. B. Saunders Co.

When A Pet Dies - A picture story for children, Fred Rogers (of Mister Rogers' Neighborhood), Harper and Row, New York, NY, 1982

When Your Pet Dies: How to Cope With Your Feelings, Jamie Quackenbush, MSW & Denise Graveline, available only through the American Animal Hospital Association, Simon & Schuster, 1985

Brochures

"Pet Loss and Bereavement," American Animal Hospital Association, Denver, CO

"Pet Loss and Human Emotion," American Veterinary Medical Association, Schaumburg, IL

Videotapes

Educational Videotape Training Program: "Pet Loss and Bereavement" - a series of three videotapes, American Animal Hospital Association, Denver, CO

"Grief From Pet Loss," Walter Weirich, DVM, Self Directed Learning Program, Stewart Center, Purdue University, West Lafayette, IN

Other Sources

The Delta Society, P.O. Box 1080, Renton, WA 98057, 206/226-7357. Publications, brochures, videotapes, names of counselors and other resource lists.

BIBLIOGRAPHY

Allen, James W., MD, MS, *Hospital Computer Systems for Health Professionals: A Cost-Benefit Approach to Assessing Alternative Technologies*, New York, NY: McGraw-Hill, Inc., 1990.

American Animal Hospital Association, *Medical Records Manual*, Denver: American Animal Hospital Association.

American Animal Hospital Association, *Standards for AAHA Hospitals*, Denver: American Animal Hospital Association.

American Veterinary Medical Association, *Marketing and Practice Strategies*, Schaumburg, Ill.: American Veterinary Medical Association, 1988.

American Veterinary Medical Association, "Principles of Veterinary Medical Ethics," *AVMA Directory*, Schaumburg, Ill.: American Veterinary Medical Association, 1991.

American Veterinary Medical Association, *Training Program for the Employees in the Veterinary Medical Practice*, Schaumburg, Ill.: American Veterinary Medical Association.

Dooley, Donald L., "The Practice Manager," *Veterinary Practice Management*, Dennis M. McCurnin, Philadelphia: J.B. Lippincott Co., 1988.

Drucker, Peter F., *The Practice of Management*, New York: Harper and Row, 1954.

Edwards, Francis G., *Marketing of Professional Services*, Tulsa, Okla.: PennWell Publishing Co., 1983.

Engel, James F., Warshaw, Martin R., Kinnear, Thomas C., *Promotional Strategy—Managing the Marketing Communications Process*, Homewood, Ill.: Irwin, 1987.

Farber, Phillip L., *History of Computers in Veterinary Practice*, The Veterinary Clinics of North America, Philadelphia: W.B. Saunders Co., July 1986.

Forney, Stuart D., "Inventory, Prescriptions and Drugs," *Veterinary Practice Management*, Dennis M. McCurnin, Philadelphia: J.B. Lippincott Co., 1988.

Friedman, Nancy, "The Telephone Doctor," Videotape #5, *Five Forbidden Phrases*, St. Louis: The Telephone Doctor.

Froehlich, Robert E., DVM, MBA, *Successful Financial Management for the Veterinary Practice*, Denver: American Animal Hospital Association, 1987.

Gaedeke, Ralph M. and Tootelian, Dennis H., *Small Business Management*, Glenview, Ill.: Scott Foresman and Co., 1985.

Gallagher, David P., *Economic and Management Considerations of a Computer*, The Veterinary Clinics of North America, Philadelphia: W.B. Saunders Co., July 1986.

Garbarino, John B., MBA, JD, *Management of the Enterprise* (Mgt. 501) lecture notes, Long Island University, Westchester Campus, Fall 1984.

Harvard Business Review, Cambridge, Mass.: Volume 66, Number 3.

Hersey, Paul and Blanchard, Ken, *Management of Organizational Behavior*, Englewood Cliffs, NJ: Prentice Hall, 4th Edition, 1982.

Hopkins, Alton F., DVM, "Pet Death: Effects on the Client and the Veterinarian," *The Pet Connection*, Minneapolis: University of Minnesota, 1984.

Internal Revenue Service, *Internal Revenue Service Code*, Reg.1.446-1(a)(1), 1986.

Lagoni, Laurel S., Arguello, Suzanne, Withrow, Stephen J. and Pike, Connee, "Patient Death and Dying," Dennis M. McCurnin, *Veterinary Practice Management*, Philadelphia: J.B. Lippincott Co., 1988.

London, Sheldon I., *How to Comply With Federal Employee Laws*, Revised Edition, Washington DC: London Publishing Company Inc., 1991.

McCafferty, Owen E., CPA, "Computers: Luxury or Necessity?" *Veterinary Economics Magazine*, March 1989.

McCulloch, William F., DVM, MPH, *The Veterinarian's Education About the Human-Animal Bond and Animal Facilitated Therapy*, The Veterinary Clinics of North America, Vol 15, No 2, Philadelphia: W.B. Saunders Co., March 1985.

McCurnin, Dennis M., DVM, *Veterinary Practice Management*, Philadelphia: J.B. Lippincott Co., 1988.

Meigs, Walter B. and Meigs, Robert F., *Financial Accounting*, fourth edition, New York: McGraw-Hill Book Company, 1986.

Murray-Hicks, Margo, *Marketing Basics for Small Entrepreneurs*, lecture presented at Training '88 Conference, N.Y.C., N.Y., December 1988, Oakland: Margo Murray-Hicks and Assoc., 1988.

Oberst, Byron B. and Long, John M., *Computers in Private Practice Management*, New York, NY: Springer-Verlag, 1987.

Schapiro, Marc, BS, MBA, *Inventory Control and Management*, lecture notes from American Animal Hospital Association Annual Meeting, Phoenix, March 1987.

Shaw, Donald R., *Your Small Business Computer: Evaluating, Selecting, Financing, Installing and Operating Hardware and Software That Fits*, New York, NY: Van Nostrand Reinhold Co., 1981.

Sheridan, John P. and McCafferty, Owen E., *The Business of Veterinary Practice*, Terrytown, NY: Pergamon Press, 1993.

Stockner, Priscilla, MS, DVM, MBA, *A Practice Management Manual for Veterinarians*, Lake San Marcos, Calif.: Stockner and Associates, 1983.

Taylor, David H., *Effects of Computers on the Practice*, The Veterinary Clinics of North America, Philadelphia: W.B. Saunders Co., July 1986.

TRENDS magazine, "Inventory Control Equals Hidden Profit," Vol.3, No.2, Denver: American Animal Hospital Association, April 1987.

Tannenbaum, Jerold, MA, JD, *Veterinary Ethics*, Baltimore: Williams and Wilkins, 1989.

Wilson, James F., DVM, JD, *Law and Ethics of the Veterinary Profession*, Yardley, Penn.: Priority Press Ltd., 1988.

Wise, J. Karl, PhD and Jih-Jing, PhD, *Computer Use and Applications in Veterinary Medicine*, Journal of the American Veterinary Medical Association, Schaumburg, Ill: The American Veterinary Medical Association, 1992.